Hair Restoration

How I restored my hair at no cost

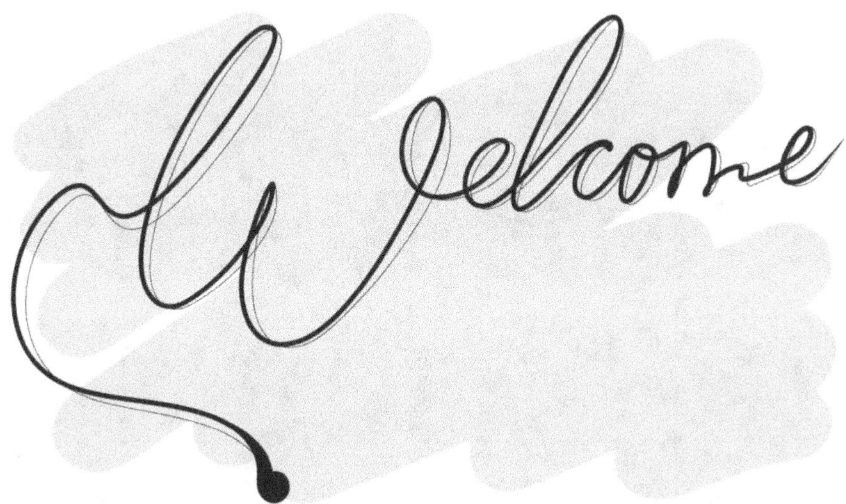

Illustrated story

Julia Moshack

Book Cover design and Illustrations by Julia Moshack
Editing and proofreading by Chris McDonalds

Thank you!

There are many ways to say "Thank you!" to other people. And I believe these simple words told to express the power of your gratitude – maybe one of the best.

Thank you very much for reading this book! I hope you'll find what you are looking for – the easy way of your hair restoration. I did all my best to describe the whole system how to make your hair grow and look wonderful again. I also created illustrations to be clear and to add some mood.

Despite of having here my recipes, my vision, and my story the book may never been published without other people.

My husband Nick Moshack was the first reader who inspired me do ahead.

My dear friends, who read the book in my native language gave me a great power to move on. Olga Lobinceva, Inga Ponomarenko, Aloina Gorodetskaya, Angel Lili Kostova, Victoria Islanova, and Zaurbeck Mizambekov – thank you so much!

The Power and Beauty of English was brought by amazing Chris McDonald. He turned my text to masterpiece. And I hope you will enjoy the language beauty as I do. Thank you a lot, Chris!

So, it's time to go :)

Table of contents

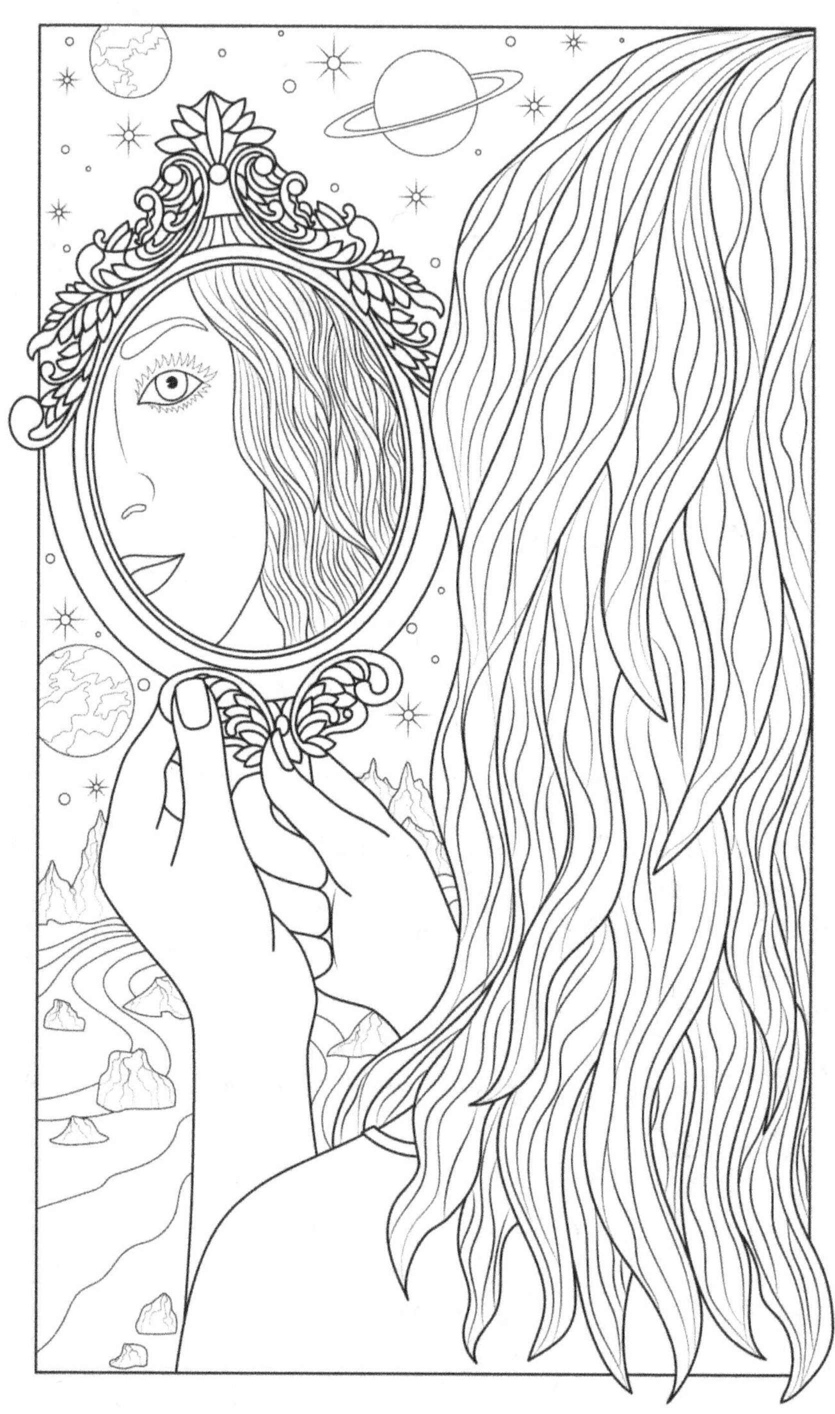

Introduction

The origins of why humans evolved to have body hair, who first proposed this idea, and the exact timing of this evolutionary development continue to be enigmatic. Yet we have grown so accustomed to these peculiar strands protruding from various parts of ourselves that the thought of parting with them—especially those that cover a significant portion of our heads—is unbearable. Some people spend years lamenting their hair's color, curl, or density, treating it like a neglected dog, subjecting it to an array of so-called miracle treatments, dyes, and devices better suited to a medieval torture chamber.

However, when our hair begins to shed like yellow autumn leaves, our sorrow knows no bounds. In desperation, we turn to any means to preserve what remains or, at the very least, create the illusion of a lush mane. Yet no matter how skillfully you arrange them, you cannot craft a beautiful lawn from three blades of grass.

I, like many, have been swept up in the tide of "investing money in my head"—or more accurately, in my hair. I have spent considerable sums on an assortment of hair care products, styling tools that momentarily allowed me to assume a different identity, and regular visits to the hairdresser for coloring and cuts. Initially, my interest was purely in the pursuit of beauty, as I understood it.

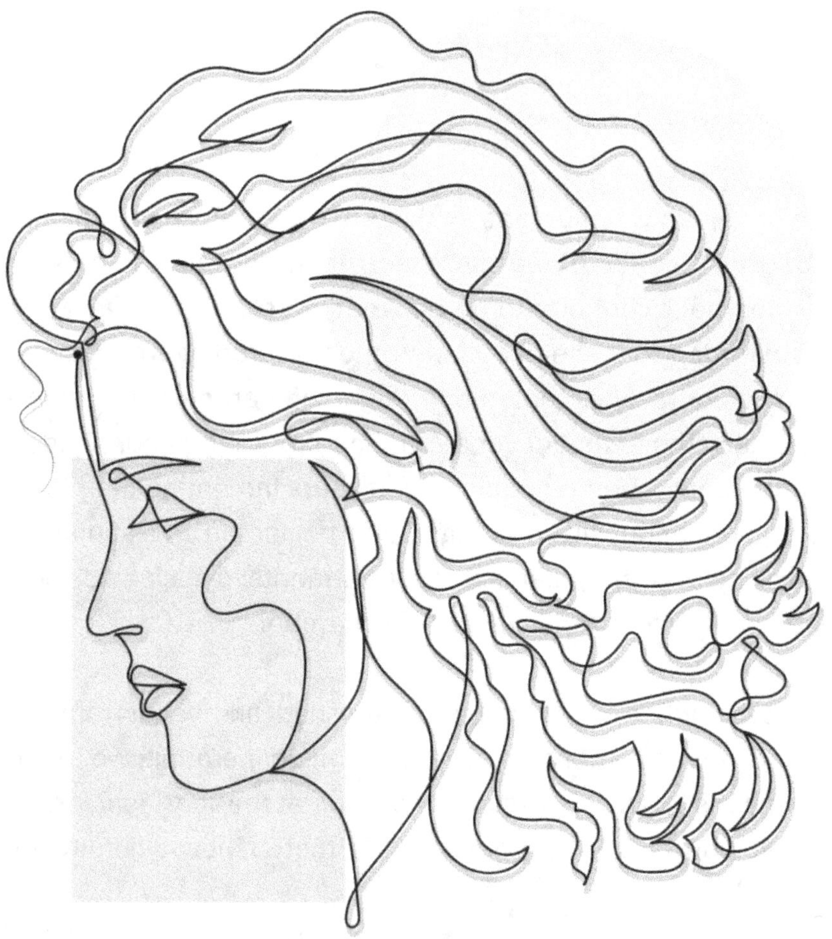

Throughout my life, I have both lost and regained my hair, although not by conscious effort. It seemed to happen of its own accord. The continual use of dyes in the quest for aesthetic enhancement eventually led to the onset of gray hairs, making coloring a necessity rather than a vanity. Have you ever noticed how humans have expanded the notion of "necessity" to almost cosmic proportions? At some juncture, I found myself contemplating such profound issues and facing decisive choices. Here's a spoiler: much of what we consider necessary is not.

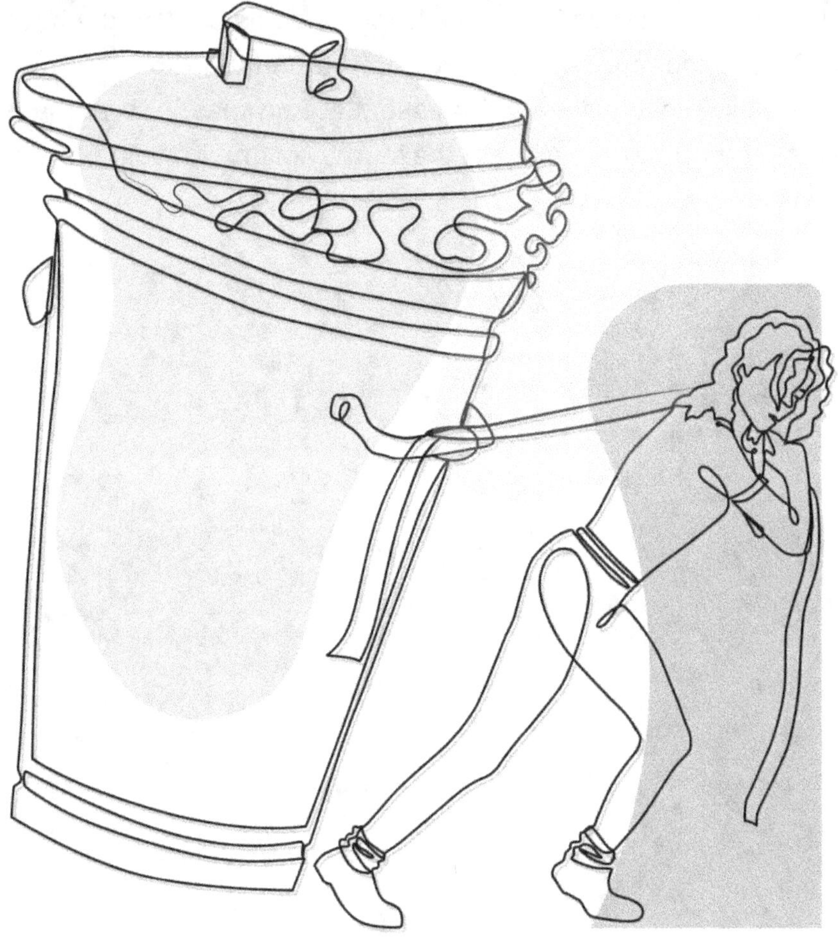

In this story, I will share with you a modest miracle that you can perform for yourself. I'll endeavor to spare you an excess of personal anecdotes, although they are, alas, inescapable. You'll discover that even if you've lost more than half your hair, a path to restoration exists. I've walked it. And it was surprisingly straightforward. So much so that I was astounded by the lack of documentation. After exhaustive research in every language I'm acquainted with, I found only sparse and scattered references.

Thus, I invite you to recline comfortably and accompany me, step by step, on this journey. I am writing this book in the hope that my experiences may serve as a foundation for your own triumphs, providing you with essential formulas, and perhaps even a complete system. Let the journey of growth begin...

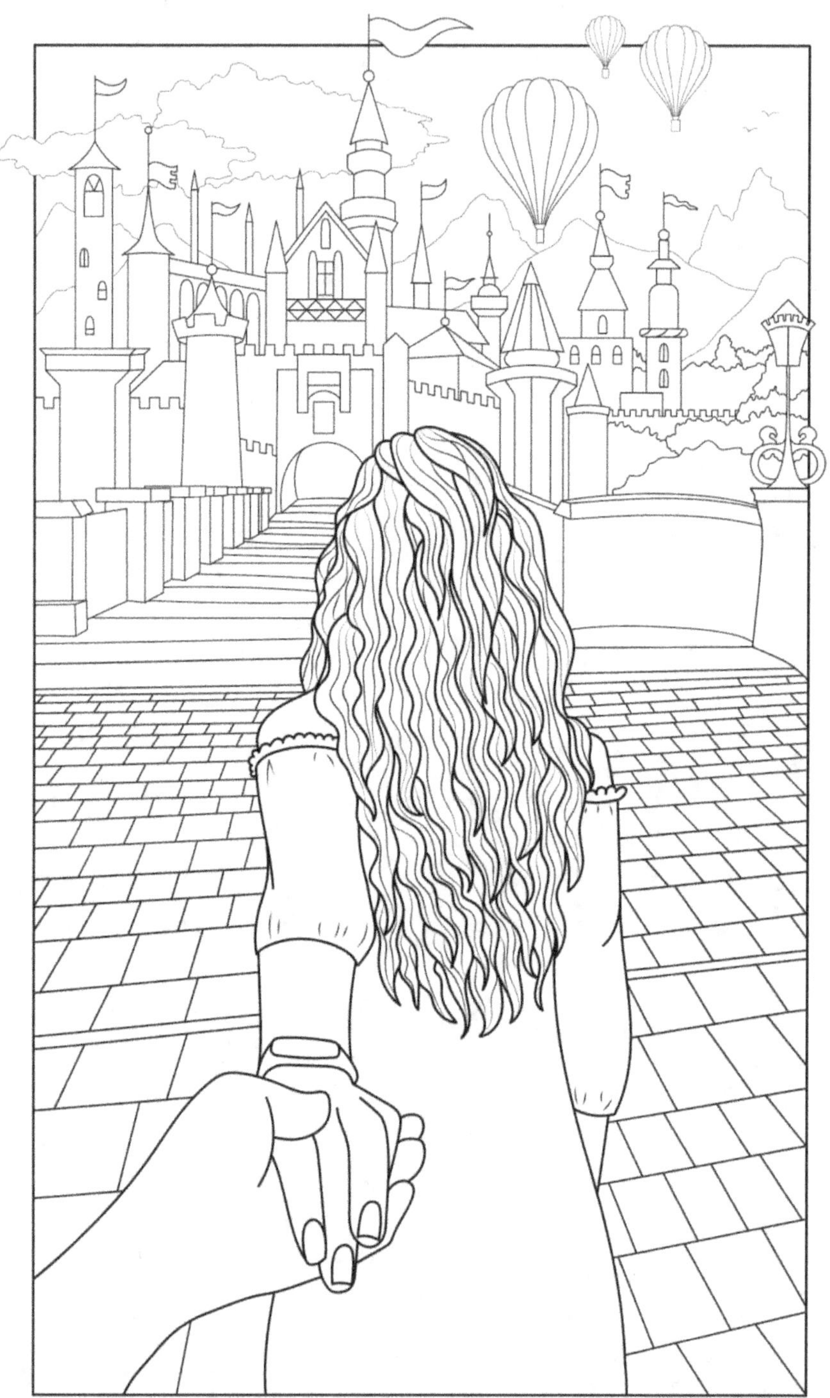

The Main Formula

Before delving into the core of my method, it's essential to outline the motivations that propelled me on this journey. Initiating this discourse is challenging, as it stirs a torrent of memories and the attendant emotions, pulling me into the past, away from the immediacy of my computer and keyboard. The term 'stress' seems too mild to encapsulate the trials I've endured. The life of every Ukrainian, particularly since February 24, 2022, could fill volumes. To spare you an inundation of details, I'll simply disclose that I nearly lost all my family and was forced to bid farewell to all my material possessions.

War's eruption unexpectedly thrust my husband and I into Europe. Bereft of plans, we had nothing but a car and a handful of belongings. To our surprise, English was not as universally spoken in Europe as we'd anticipated, which compounded the challenges of finding shelter, managing registrations, and learning the ropes—all while grappling with a new language. I felt utterly out of my element. The distressing news from Ukraine plunged me into despair, and personal losses made me forget how to breathe, how to live.

Adding to this was the startling revelation that food tastes different abroad, not always aligning with our palates. Fast food became a dubious sanctuary, but such a diet hardly promotes health. Despite these hardships, we were fortunate. Kind-hearted people from various countries extended their help, earning my eternal gratitude.

Fleeing the agony my homeland had transformed into, we found refuge in Portugal, the so-called "End of the World," for several months. Eventually, we moved to Bulgaria, seeking a climate and cuisine that echoed home. Slowly, life began to regain semblance, allowing me to shift focus from existential pain to more mundane concerns, like my hair. From here on, our narrative turns away from sorrow to the topic at hand: hair restoration.

The factors of stress, diet, climate, inconsistent care, and varying hairdressers and dyes, unsurprisingly, don't foster hair retention. My hair began to abandon its roots in protest.

The remnants of this exodus were stark against my floor—dark, long strands that told of my strife. The gray hairs that had infiltrated my once-uniform color necessitated increasingly frequent dyeing, and the realization that I had lost half of my hair volume compounded my worry. Yet, what troubled me most was the burgeoning gray. I grew weary of constant coloring, but the idea of revealing my graying reality to the world was unthinkable at the time.

Thus began my research on gray hair. The consensus among experts was discouraging, asserting that reversing graying was an impossibility. Weary of fretting over the inevitable, I decided to take action.

The premise I adopted was uncomplicated, and the ensuing actions, even more so. After six months, I rejoiced in the resurgence of my hair—thicker, with new growth. The gray hair issue persisted, as I continued to color it, making it difficult to assess that particular aspect.

Here lies the crux of my approach:

The essential equation: ***Good hair = blood * time***

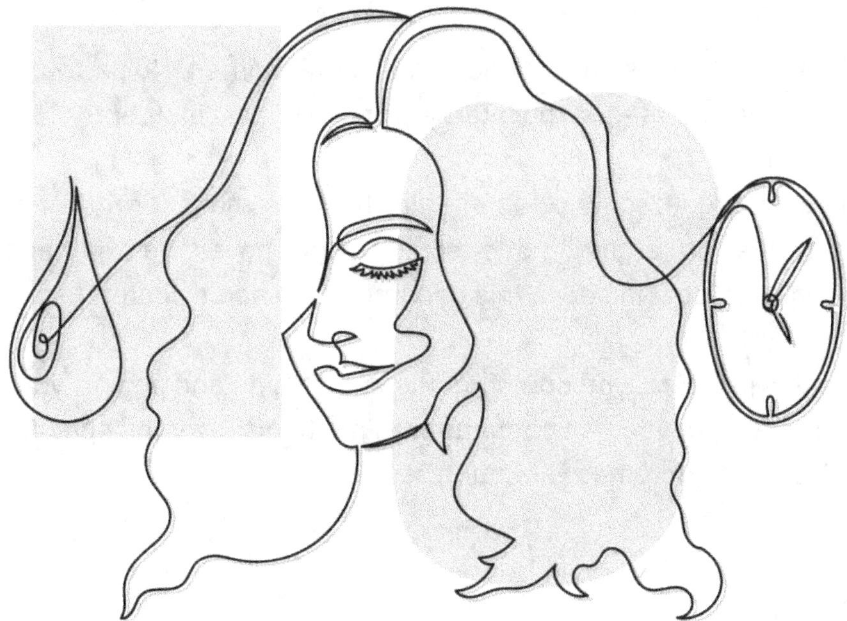

Now, let's liken hair to a plant.

For a plant to thrive from a seed, it requires nutrient-rich soil. Without these nutrients, growth is doubtful. And what transports nutrients to every cell your body? Precisely, blood. I needed to increase blood circulation to the scalp, enriching my hair with the requisite sustenance.

Like plants, hair growth is not an overnight phenomenon (growing only about 1 to 1.5 centimeters monthly), and some hair may enter a dormant phase, much like hibernating bears. Have you ever roused a bear from hibernation? I haven't, though it's theoretically possible. The bear analogy is a digression, intended to paint the broader picture. I gave myself a six-month timeline, reasoning that anticipating results any sooner was futile. It was purely experimental, with no room for premature despair.

These two points are the backbone of my regimen. No profound mysteries here—just the interplay of two critical elements.

Life, I've realized, is often simpler than we make it out to be, solvable with a couple of straightforward moves. Yet, humans relish secrets, and now, this becomes our shared secret :)

At this juncture, you could put the guide aside and ponder your approach, or you can continue with me to discover the specific ideas and outcomes I encountered.

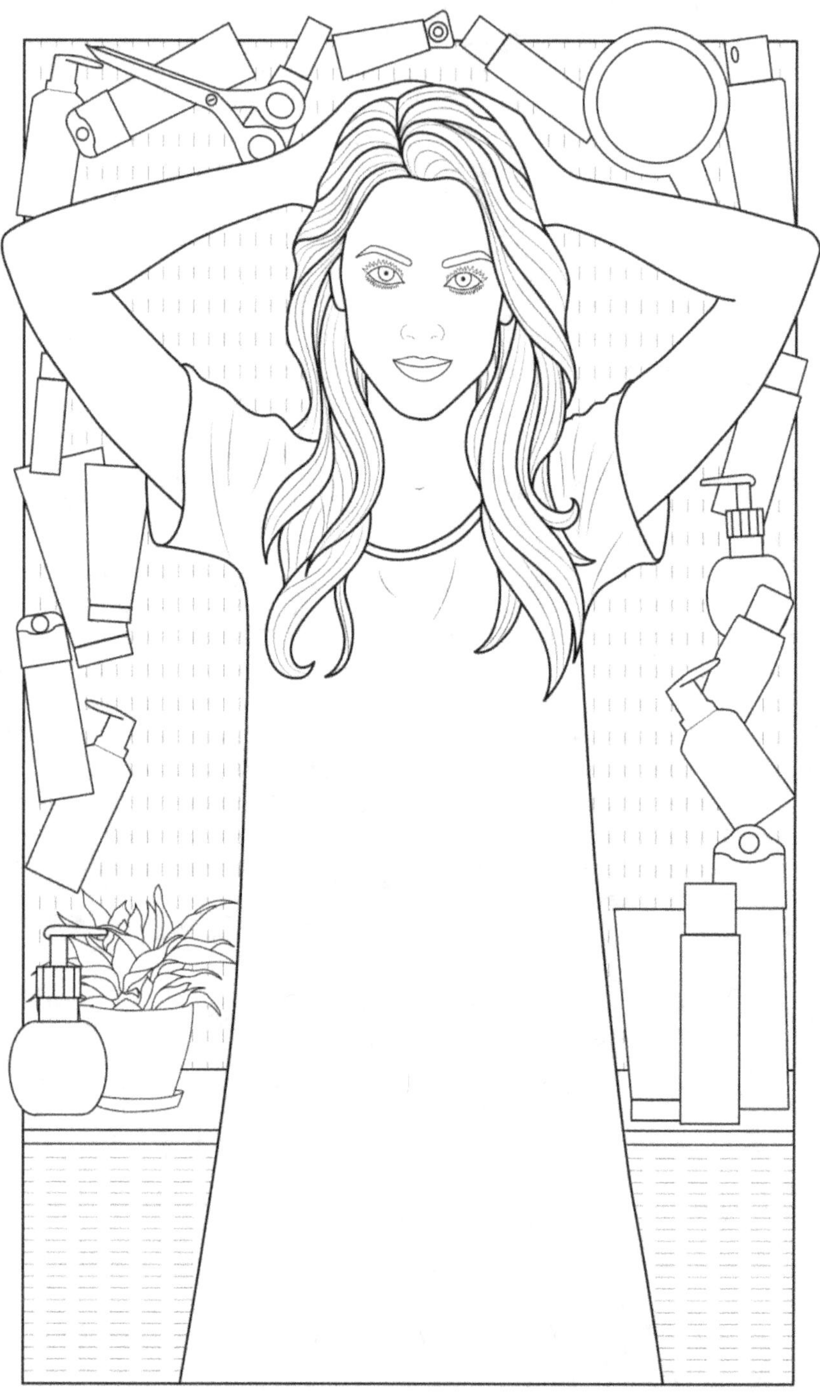

My Actions

Acknowledging the need for increased blood flow to the hair roots set the stage for my action plan. Contemplating the "how," I considered various methods: inversion postures, stimulating scalp rubs with spices like pepper or onion, or purchasing specialized treatments designed to enhance circulation.

Yet, my aim was simplicity and self-reliance, seeking something secure, effortless, affordable, and independent. My talented Kyiv hairdresser was irreplaceable, and as life's unpredictability could lead me anywhere, I aspired for a method impervious to changes in location or professionals.

Thus, the solution was evident—self-massage of the scalp. Simple in theory, yet challenging in practice, as effective self-massage demands considerable hand and finger strength, which I lacked. This need for physical robustness might explain why, despite abundant online endorsements of scalp massages, testimonials of actual success are scarce.

Lacking the necessary strength, yet undeterred, I turned to a regular massage hairbrush.

Taking the First Steps

I would like to express a concern that you might interpret the guidance I'm about to provide too literally, which could lead to discomfort on your part. You also might wonder about my investment in this matter. Well, I value comfort quite highly and fully understand the importance of the care and attention we lavish upon ourselves. This philosophy has guided my journey, one I have paced deliberately and enjoyed immensely. Thus, I am willing to make a suggestion: act within the limits of your comfort. Use my method as a source of inspiration, adapting it to fit your needs so that it suits you just right.

My routine began with a simple activity: brushing my hair 100 times, switching the direction with each stroke. When one hand became weary, I would switch to the other.

To prevent the task from becoming tedious, I added gentle movements to the rhythm of brushing, akin to a dance – swaying my hips to the right and left, also 100 times. This turned the process into a mini exercise session, and I suspect that enhancing blood circulation plays a part in achieving desired outcomes.

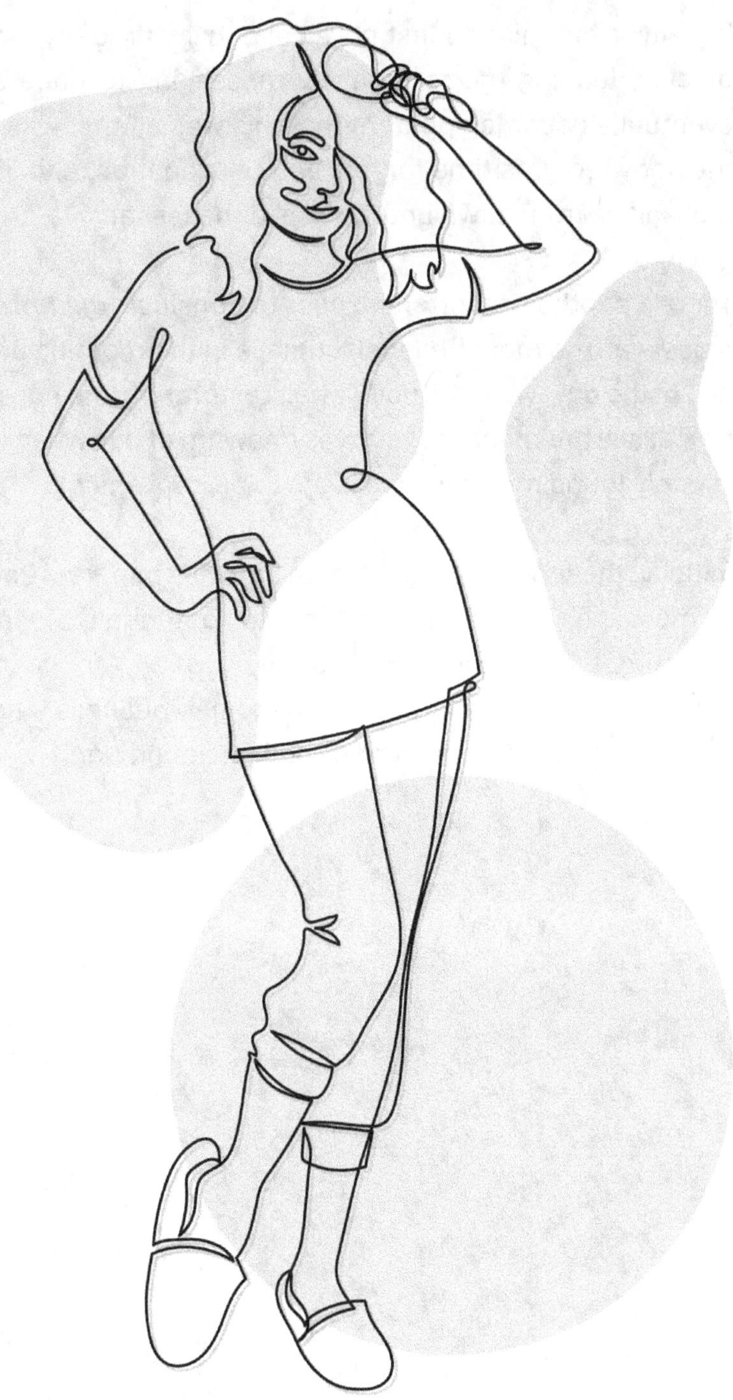

Initially, even this modest physical activity tired my arms quite quickly, leading me to limit my massaging to once a day. It eventually became apparent that this was all that was needed; the body requires time for rest and rejuvenation, and incessant massaging from dawn until dusk is unnecessary.

There's another important aspect to consider: *the timing of the massage*. The most beneficial time is in the morning or the first half of the day when the body's hair restoration and nourishment processes are most active. I was unaware of this when I started; I simply found morning massages to be convenient.

Initially, the process took no more than five minutes. Performing a massage in the evening could potentially lead to an overstimulated nervous system, which is particularly unwelcome if one is already prone to nervousness. There is no sense in aggravating an already delicate condition.

Initial Challenges

The adoption of my new regimen yielded results almost instantly, albeit not the ones I had anticipated. My hair began to shed significantly, which naturally caused me distress. The urge to abandon the process was strong. Nonetheless, my resolve to adhere to the six-month plan was my saving grace, so I persisted.

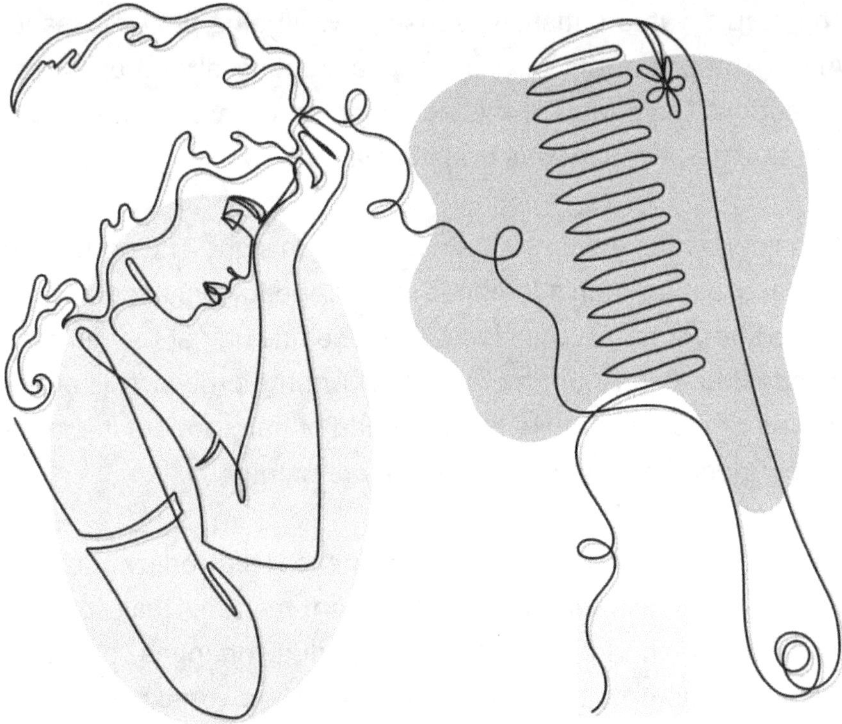

In an effort to decipher the cause of my hair's reaction, I dived into the depths of the Internet. It didn't take long to find several sources confirming that my experience was normal. My hair shedding intensified, but this is a typical response. I will delve into the reasons for this in the "A bit of Theory" section.

Emerging Delights

Gradually, both my hands and scalp grew stronger. I began to brush my hair 200, then 300 times, using a different brush for each set of a hundred strokes. I owned three. This variety made my "dance" movements during the process more complex, and each set of strokes was paired with its own unique motion.

The result was a satisfying sense of wellbeing post-massage. About three months in, I noticed a curious alteration in my reflection. The shape of my face seemed different – it was my hair that had wrought this transformation!

Consider a man losing his hair: a common sight. The hair at the center of such a man's forehead often appears longer compared to the shorter hair at the sides. The receding hair at the temples invades the fuller hair, marching toward the crown. This effect can be present in men with a full head of hair too, but it's more pronounced and stark in those who are balding.

The reason for sharing this is the unexpected realization that women could experience a similar phenomenon. Daily scrutiny in the mirror hadn't revealed any gradual changes, as I had grown accustomed to my reflection. Then, unexpectedly, I observed a shift. My left hairline, changing from square to an oval shape, echoed the hairline of my youth. On the right, the hair was only beginning to grow back, allowing me to see both square and oval shapes simultaneously. Quite the spectacle, indeed! But, it was, of course, a welcome sign of progress. Patience was all that was needed now.

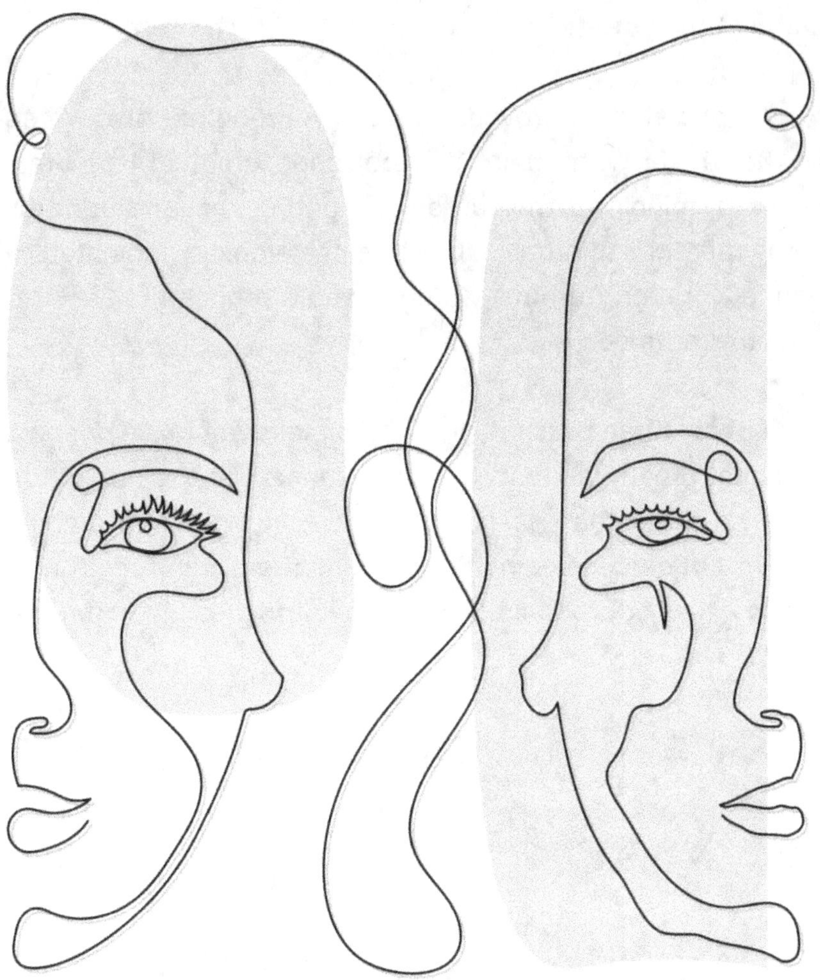

This was when I grasped that people striving for a youthful look often concentrate on superficial solutions. Cosmetics and surgery are not panaceas. A youthful demeanor consists of subtle details: the skin's health, the contour of the forehead (a young forehead, in profile, lacks fleshiness and has clean, smooth lines), one's posture and walk, animated facial expressions, the capacity for wonder, and a twinkle in the eye. I had not anticipated that the hairline would join this list, but the difference it made was clear. The discovery left me in awe.

Refining the System

As my proficiency improved, so did my strength. I discovered that 100 strokes with a hairbrush took approximately 4 minutes. To ease my mind from the burden of counting, I began setting my watch timer for 5 minutes. Once the time elapsed, indicated by a gentle vibration from my watch, I would proceed to the next part of my routine.

Not all of my three brushes provided a pleasurable experience. The oldest brush had lost the small spheres at the tips of the bristles, a detail that wasn't noticeable during short combing sessions but became painfully apparent after 5 minutes. Thus, I devised a new approach: using only two brushes but in a novel manner.

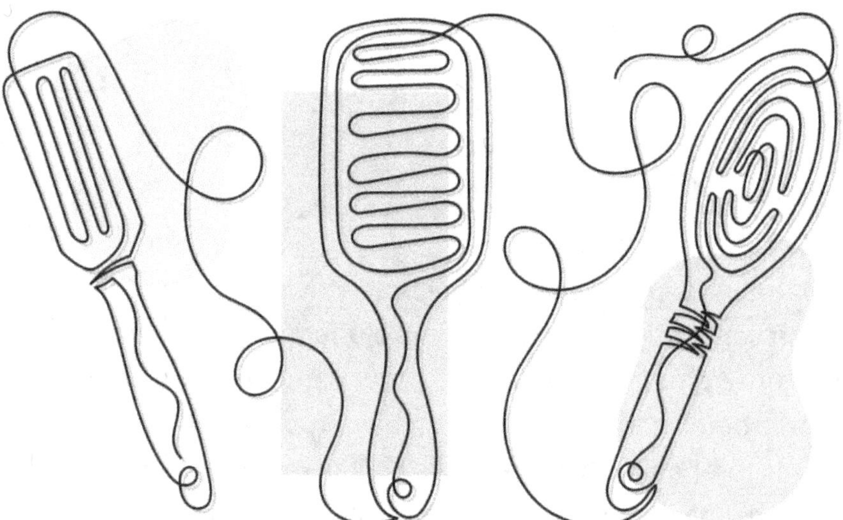

I retained the initial phase of my routine—5 minutes of brushing in various directions with one brush. However, in the second phase, I introduced my new soft, wide brush as the centerpiece.

This brush, covering a broad swath of my scalp, ensures no harm to the skin. I adopted it primarily for massaging.
While it would be easiest to show you the technique in person, given the distance, I will attempt to illustrate the process in words, supplemented by images, acknowledging the adage that a picture is worth a thousand words.

The first step is massaging the hairline with the soft, wide hairbrush. I place the brush against my forehead, ensuring that the majority of its surface contacts the scalp, with a portion on the skin. The objective is to massage areas near the hairline, vital for blood circulation. I initiate with gentle circular motions, applying slight pressure to warm up the scalp. I haven't timed this precisely; it's about 3 to 5 seconds. Following this brief massage, I glide the brush to the right or left, maintaining the circular motion, circling back to my starting point.

Noticing that the crown of the head often gets neglected, I methodically massage every section with the same circular motions, beginning near an ear and parting the hair in sections, moving towards the opposite ear, and then back again.
The massage concludes in the same fashion it began, with circular strokes along the hair growth line. On average, this whole procedure takes between 15 to 20 minutes.

That encapsulates the complete system. When I had tailored it to my liking, I contemplated increasing the massage duration or intensity. Eventually, I concluded there was no need for further modifications as they would not yield additional benefits. Instead, I opted to allocate my newfound time and strength to other engaging pursuits.

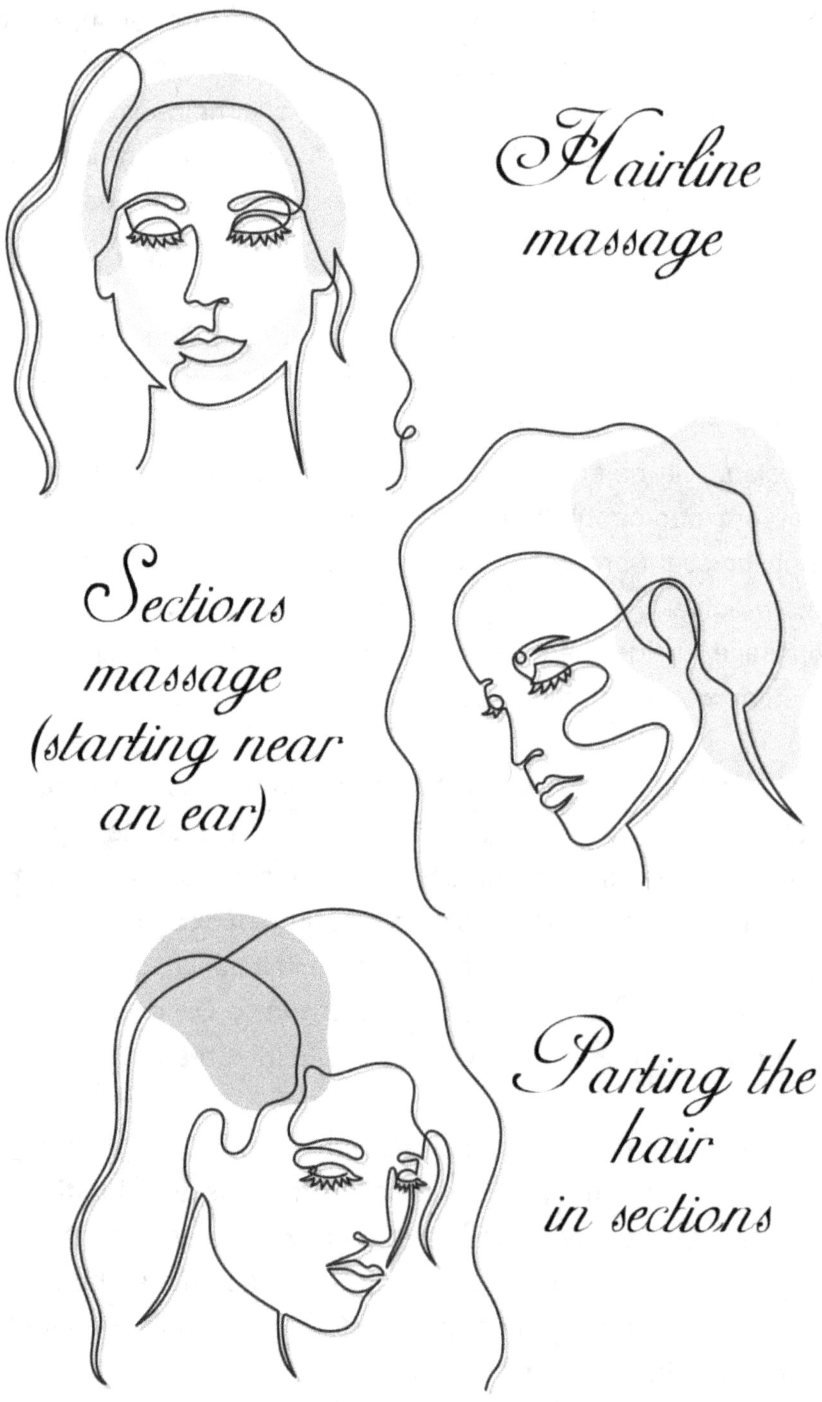
Hairline massage
Sections massage (starting near an ear)
Parting the hair in sections

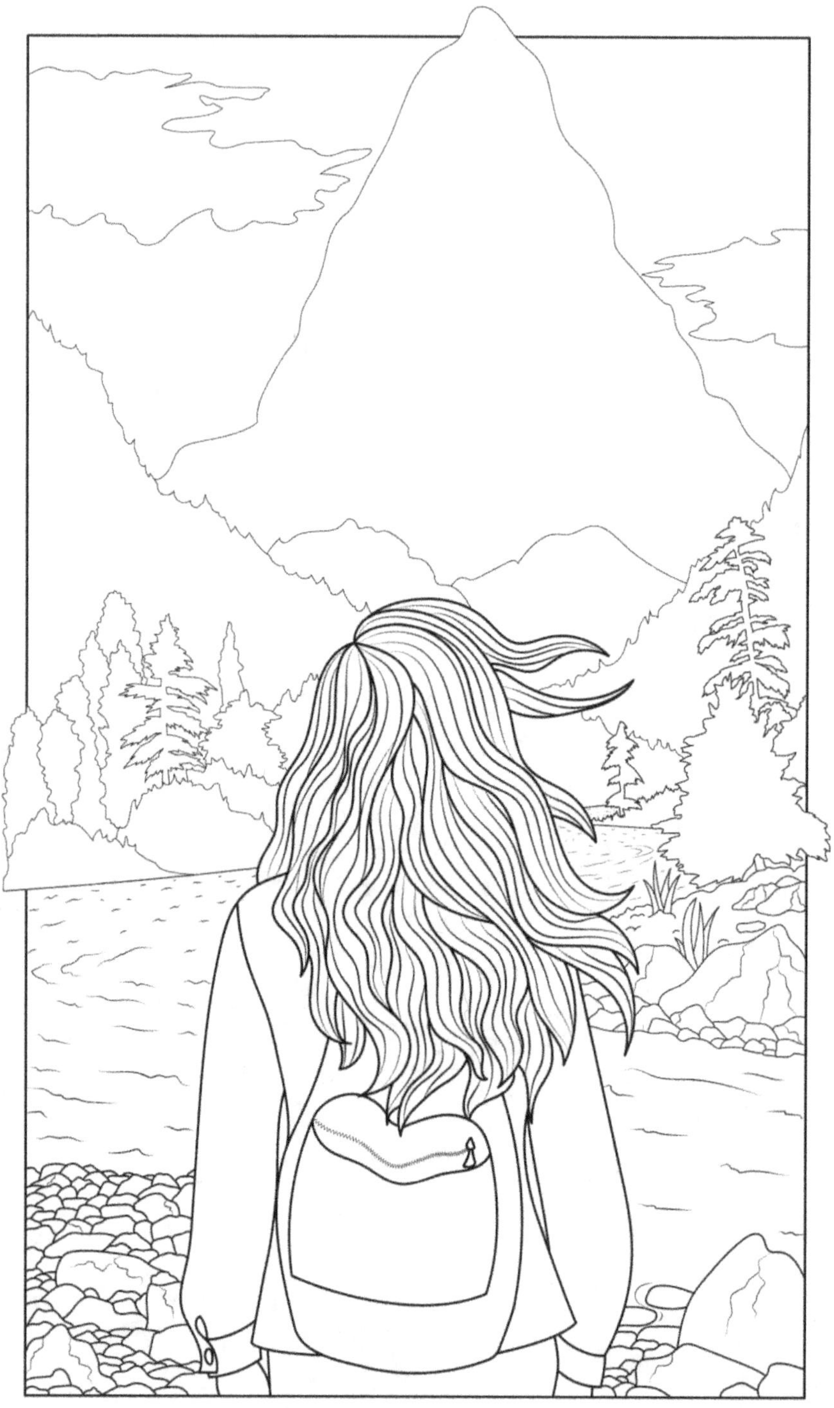

Main Challenges

Every journey is bound to encounter unexpected developments, not all of which are welcome. Recognizing this, I resolved to consider what prompted reflection and the need for new decisions.

As I've noted before, I experienced a noticeable increase in hair loss during the initial couple of months. This is a typical response; the key is to endure this phase.

My hairbrushes required more frequent cleaning as they accumulated dirt faster, but these are minor inconveniences in the grand scheme of things.

An unexpected occurrence was the development of a rash on my scalp, a sign that the skin was reacting to the stimulation and the cleansing of pores—a natural aspect of the process. In my experience, it was a minor issue. I occasionally noticed small rashes, but they vanished swiftly and did not recur. However, it's advisable to refrain from touching affected areas until they heal. I will not belabor the importance of medical consultation for serious conditions, as it goes without saying.

I recently watched a video featuring a man attempting to regrow hair on his extensively bald scalp using a massage device. His diligence was laudable, but his technique was confounding. He vigorously massaged his scalp multiple times daily, seeking rapid growth. Ready to commit months to this regimen, he nonetheless inflicted excessive distress upon himself, creating abrasions in pursuit of stimulating hair growth, without considering the potential harm.

Transforming a soothing scalp massage into a painful ordeal is unnecessary. Yet, it seems a prevailing belief that beauty is worth such personal sacrifice. This individual, despite enduring pain and injury, was steadfast in his journey toward an envisioned future. He showcased photos before and after four months of treatment, revealing some progress. However, the outcome might have been improved had he adopted a more moderate approach. It begs reflection: if the body is dealing with wounds, it prioritizes healing over hair growth, redirecting resources accordingly.

Through reflection and experimentation, I've come to understand that our bodies are remarkably responsive. If we guide them with a gentle, consistent, and deliberate approach towards an attainable goal, success is within our reach, all without subjecting ourselves to harsh treatments and while enjoying the journey. This realization prompted another significant life decision.

Previously, I regularly visited the hairdresser to dye my hair and conceal the grey strands. An unforgettable incident occurred during the fifth appointment following the initiation of my hair restoration regimen. As was my routine, I spent 15 to 20 minutes massaging my scalp that morning.
For those unacquainted with hair coloring, the process involves multiple steps: the application of dye, a waiting period of around 40 minutes, followed by rinsing, drying, and styling.

However, that day's experience turned disastrous. After the dye was applied, as I sat reading on my phone, a burning sensation overwhelmed my scalp. This discomfort was unexpected and severe. Hampered by a language barrier in my current country of residence, I relied on an electronic translator to convey the urgency of my situation to the hairdresser. Her nonchalance, based on the familiarity of the procedure, did little to assuage my concerns. Despite reassurances of safety, I endured the pain until it subsided. This distressing reaction, so different from previous experiences, led me to question the changes occurring within me. Why now, after so many years, was my body reacting so violently?

In any puzzling situation, seeking information is undoubtedly worthwhile. Even when bits of knowledge are dispersed across vast distances, diligent search efforts can lead to discovery. It became clear to me that my skin was rejuvenating. With gradual, incremental steps, it was healing: pores reopened, and breathability was restored. My skin's sensitivity normalized, and nerve cells resumed their crucial roles, transmitting impulses appropriately. I became attuned to these signals, gaining awareness of them. Naturally, the harsh chemicals previously used to mask my grey hair did not escape notice given this newfound sensitivity. I resolved to forgo scalp massages before hair coloring to avoid discomfort.

When the time came to act on this decision, the recovery process for my skin was already underway, gaining momentum. The sensitivity that had been dulled by past dyeing sessions was reviving, leading to a fresh bout of discomfort, albeit milder. Even with soothing oils applied by my hairdresser, the irritation persisted.

This experience prompted me to question the worth of conventional beauty rituals. The perception in my country equates grey hair on a woman with a sense of personal defeat, signaling the end of vibrancy. I had been oblivious to the option of embracing my natural hair color, my conception of beauty shaped by the standards propagated by the media. Yet, beauty is subjective—ask a dozen individuals what beauty means to them, and you'll receive a dozen different perspectives.

For the first time, I began to observe people from a new perspective, and it was as if a different world had unfolded before me — a world where grey hair was celebrated for its natural beauty. The impulse to conceal or dye it seemed pointless. Astonishingly, there's a burgeoning movement, predominantly among women, who are reclaiming their right to embrace their grey hair. This phenomenon is astonishing; in an era that boasts freedom, the ingrained stereotype is remarkably pervasive, not just in my homeland of Ukraine but globally. Individuals often go to great lengths to hide their age from themselves and others, treating it as if it were a closely guarded secret. One must wonder, do we possess a sincere explanation for this within ourselves?

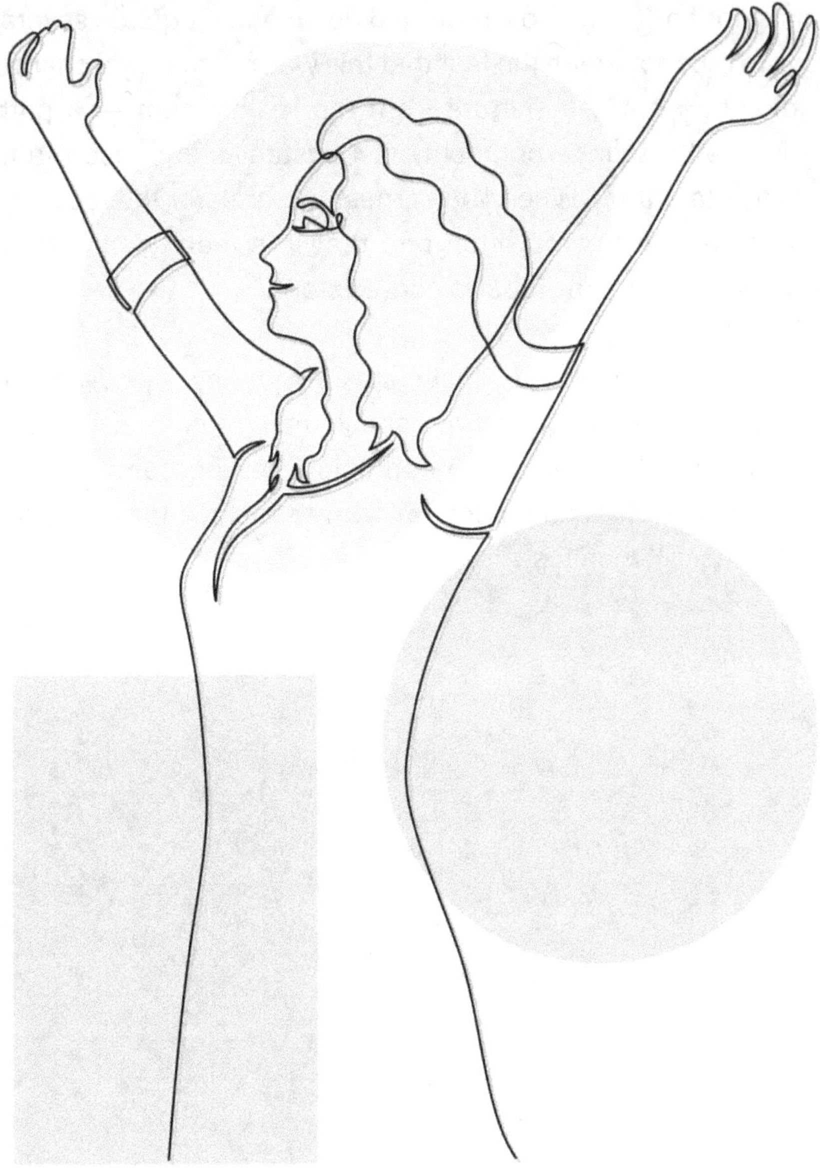

Admittedly, I was taken aback by the revelation of how deeply entrenched and unnatural these beliefs were within me, having harbored them for years without recognizing that an alternative was always evident.

This epiphany led me to a profound decision. It required several days to reconcile with the fact that this was not merely a change in direction but a departure from the mainstream — a path fraught with intense competition, constant comparison, and illusory standards. When you earnestly search for that coveted ideal to aspire to, you often find that it is merely an illusion because, in truth, the ideal is non-existent.

Looking inward poses its challenges. Regarding my hair, there remains a considerable journey ahead until my natural hair fully regrows. Yet, I've learned to appreciate the passage of time, understanding that days accumulate into years, and eventually, outcomes will manifest.

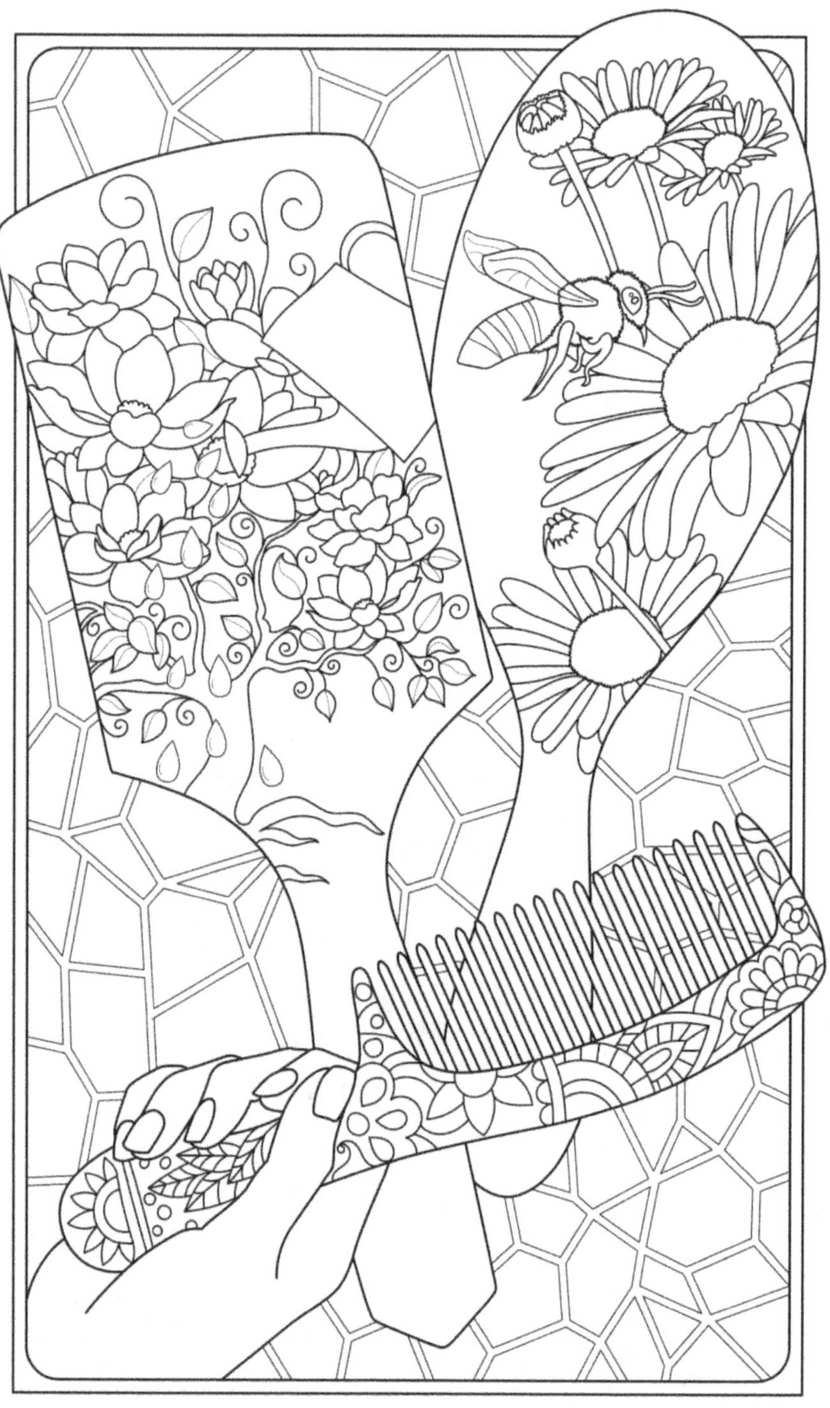

Results

At the time I composed this book, it has been eight months into my hair restoration journey. What transformations have occurred during this period?

Hair Growth: The most discernible alteration has been the substantial growth of new hair. Every parting reveals a burgeoning "forest" of hair ranging from minuscule to 6-8 centimeters. This abundance now imparts a voluminous appearance to my hair, reminiscent of my student days, a time I had almost forgotten.

In researching hair, I often encountered the notion that genetics is the ultimate determinant and that change is futile. Initially, I accepted this, thinking: "Naturally, everyone loses hair with age. Perhaps change is indeed impossible." However, witnessing the emergence of new hair, I comprehended the true meaning behind the scientists' words.

They implied that altering innate traits, like hair color or texture, is implausible, but restoring what once existed is feasible. This revelation is invigorating as it allows one to be their best, natural self.

Despite my progress, I persist with daily massages. Without hair dye, the rapid pace of hair growth became evident, especially at the temples where growth exceeded 2 centimeters in a month, and on the crown, about 1.5 cm, aligning with specialists' upper norm. Previously indifferent to the rate of hair growth, the cultivation of my natural color has now piqued my interest in it.

Increased Hand Strength: An unforeseen benefit was the strengthening of my hands, not an initial objective. Regular massaging, even with a hairbrush, necessitates hand involvement, which bolstered my strength incrementally. From an initial 4 to 5 minutes, my massage sessions can now extend to 25 minutes. This newfound strength has enabled me to undertake other exercises that require arm power and to delight in activities like facial massage.

Stronger Nails: Another surprising development was the fortification of my fingernails. This realization dawned on me five months into my hair care routine, acknowledging that the constant hand activity and consequent blood flow naturally enhance nail growth and strength.

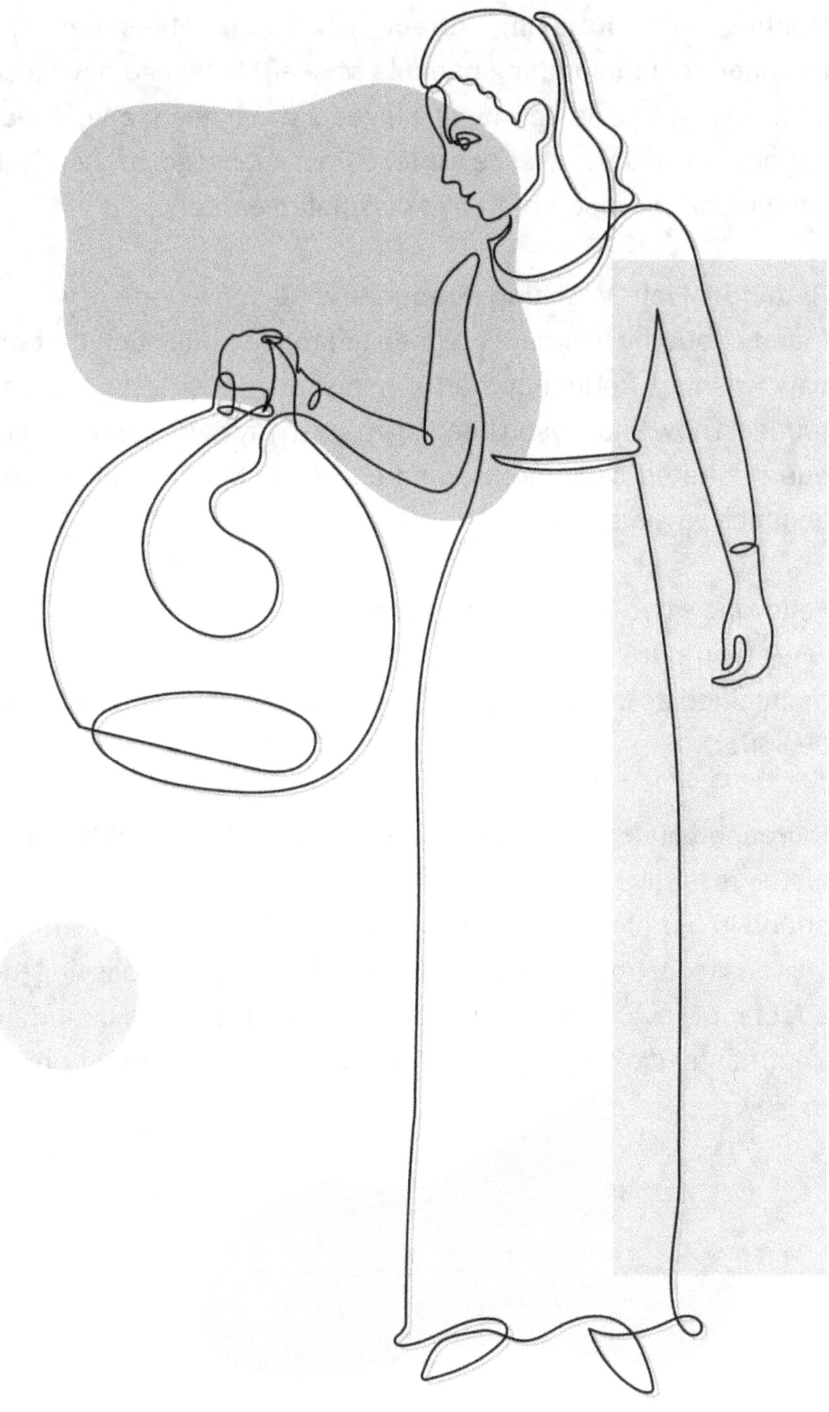

Healing and Relaxing Effect of Scalp Massage: The therapeutic and soothing benefits of scalp massage have also been evident. One morning, plagued by a headache, I was curious about the massage's effect. Post-massage, my head felt lighter, and the discomfort had dissipated entirely.

Reduced Hair Washing Frequency: A conversation with a friend about my hair care regimen led to the realization that my hair washing frequency had diminished. Previously a 3-day routine, I now find myself needing to wash my hair every 4-5 days due to altered sebaceous gland activity, which simplifies and enhances my life.

Following a two-month interval, I conducted an experiment of a week without hair washing, to surprising results. My hair maintained its freshness as though it had been washed a day or two prior.

Increased Hair Shine: Lastly, the reason behind healthy hair's luster is straightforward: sebaceous glands enshroud each strand in a protective coating, preserving moisture and vitality. This has led to my hair glistening more than ever, surpassing the effects of even the most luxurious and professional hair treatments. It's an unexpected and welcome result that brings me joy.

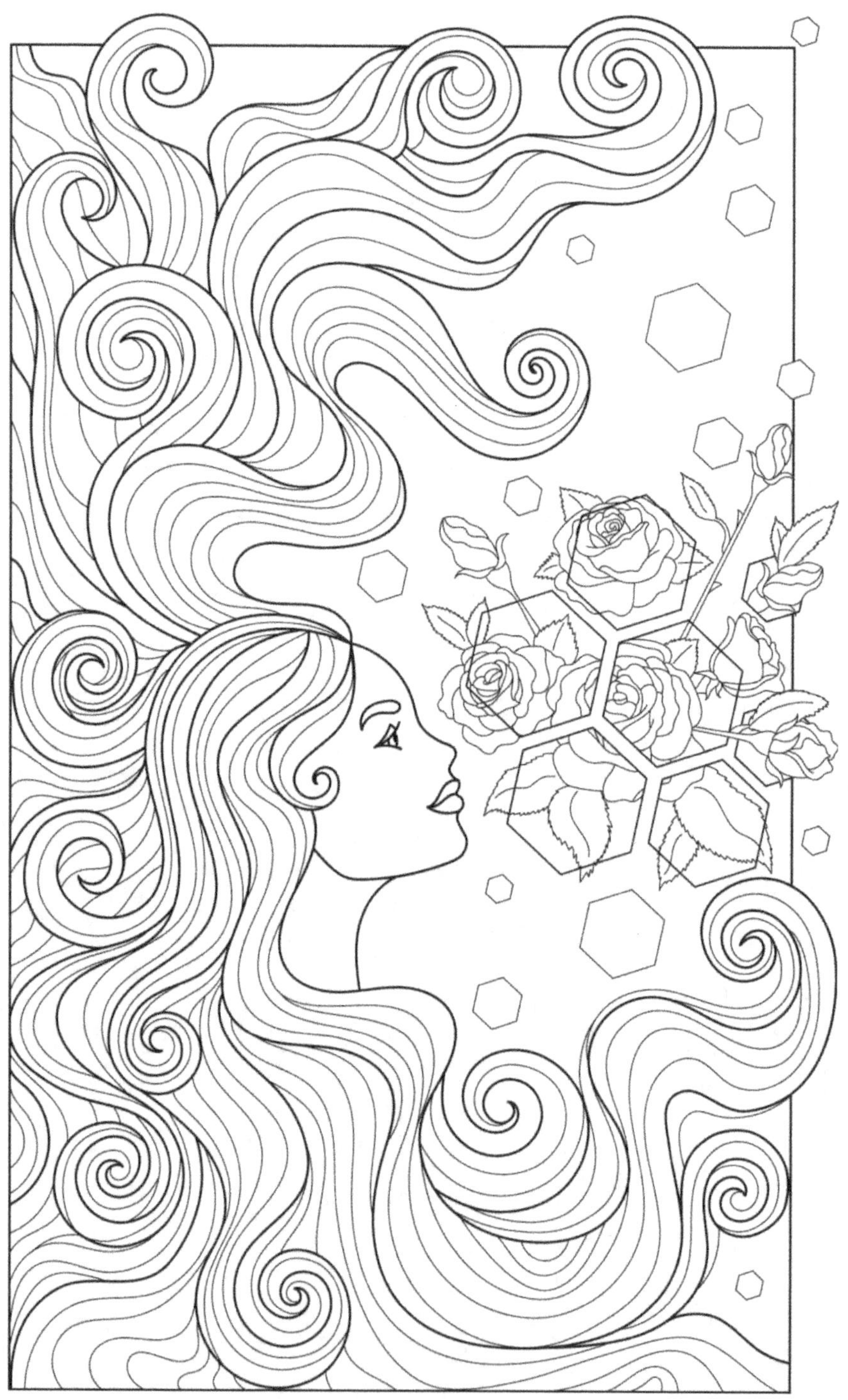

Additional Activities

I am not a medical professional, so I don't claim that all issues can be resolved as if by magic. It's plausible that factors beyond massage have contributed to the positive results I've observed. Different aspects of my lifestyle might have had a direct or indirect influence on solving a problem. Just as a painting is more than a standout brushstroke or central figure, but a tapestry of elements including the backdrop and secondary objects, everything works in concert. It only makes sense to view a part of our body in isolation if it is no longer attached. Otherwise, each hair is part of a complex system. What follows is a description of other activities that I favor and incorporate regularly.

Physical Activity: How I wish maintaining our body's prime condition was as simple as dusting off a beautiful statue occasionally. However, that's not possible—we are living beings. Our bodies need to breathe and move, and every moment there are numerous processes occurring within. Movement facilitates these processes, and each person has the autonomy to choose their preferred form of activity.

Apart from the "dancing" I do while massaging, as mentioned earlier, I engage in two other significant activities. The first is a simple exercise routine I perform at home on a yoga mat. The second is taking daily walks in the open air. When time is scarce, and someone asks about my priority, I unequivocally choose walking. Like plants, we need sunlight, even when it's obscured by clouds.

Experts recommend a minimum of 30 minutes of outdoor time daily for good health and well-being. The optimal walking pace allows for a comfortable conversation.

My initial walking speed was just 3 kilometers per hour, with frequent breaks due to my sedentary job. Now I can comfortably walk at over 6 kilometers per hour, rendering my usual routes and parks seemingly smaller. The plethora of benefits walking offers could fill volumes, but a good start involves watching a few videos on proper foot placement and simply beginning to walk.

The preference for other physical exercises or sports varies by individual. Personally, I've never been sporty, which led to repeated failures in athletic endeavors until I ceased the struggle with my body. I questioned what I enjoyed most and found joy in stretching, an activity I truly love.

Water: Indeed, humans are predominantly water-based. Vital processes, including hair growth, are dependent on water. Therefore, emulating a flowing stream rather than a stagnant swamp is beneficial. I drink a substantial amount of water, particularly in the morning. Through experimentation, I've learned how my body responds to hydration and prefer it well-hydrated.

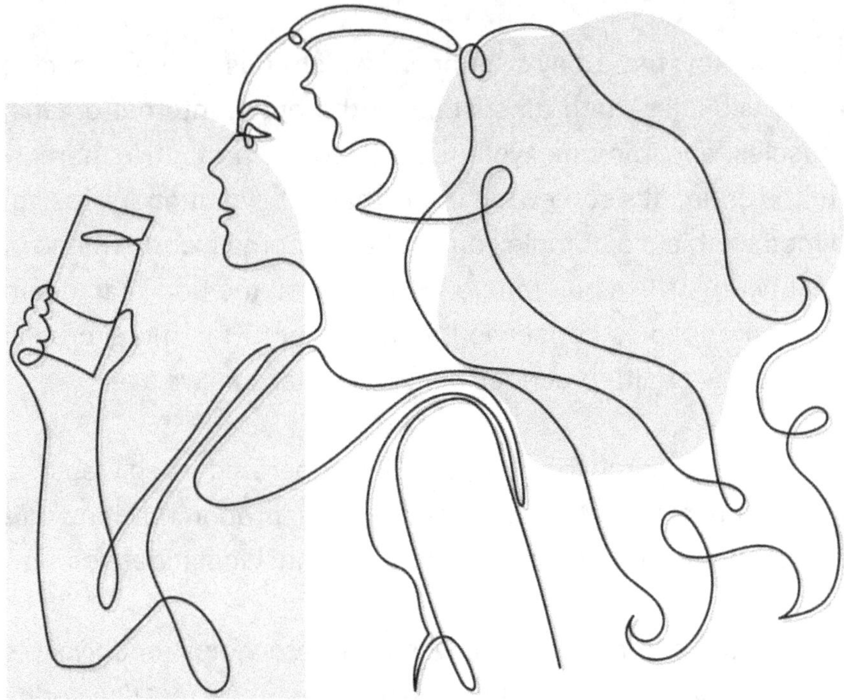

I refrain from dictating a specific water intake as individual needs vary, influenced by factors like genetics, sex, weight, height, age, and climate. Starting with general World Health Organization recommendations, I began to tailor my hydration practices. Drinking water has become an essential daily habit for me, one that I track with a to-do list on my phone, marking it off once I've consumed the necessary amount each day.

Nutrition: In the beginning, when I highlighted the importance of blood and its role in transporting nutrients, I did not elaborate on the origins of these nutrients—sourced from water, food, and air (hence, the significance of walks).
I dedicated time to discern the types of food conducive to promoting healthy hair growth. Amidst a wealth of information, I found only nuggets of wisdom.

Hair is not the body's priority, which has more pressing responsibilities such as sustaining the brain, internal organs, muscles, and immune system. Hair's role is protective, namely for the brain. (It's somewhat ironic that our evolutionary design, aimed to shield a complex organ, has become a centerpiece of beauty rituals like hair rollers.) For survival, the body can deem hair expendable, conserving vital nutrients for more crucial functions—health precedes hair, particularly as we age.

I ceased my search for a hair-specific superfood when I realized that none exists. The true 'secrets' to proper nutrition are apparent and simple: provide the body with what it desires.

My approach to food shopping is exploratory, as if each visit is my first. I aim to be receptive to what I genuinely feel like eating at the moment. Occasionally, my choices may appear unusual, but I steer clear of processed and semi-processed foods. I focus primarily on healthy options, mindful that our stomach's capacity is finite and the body requires a rich array of nutrients. Hence, it's unwise to consume non-nutritive substances. The foundational principles of my diet are timeless: 25% protein (vital for hair health), 25% carbohydrates, and 50% fruits and vegetables—nothing outlandish, just the essence of simplicity.

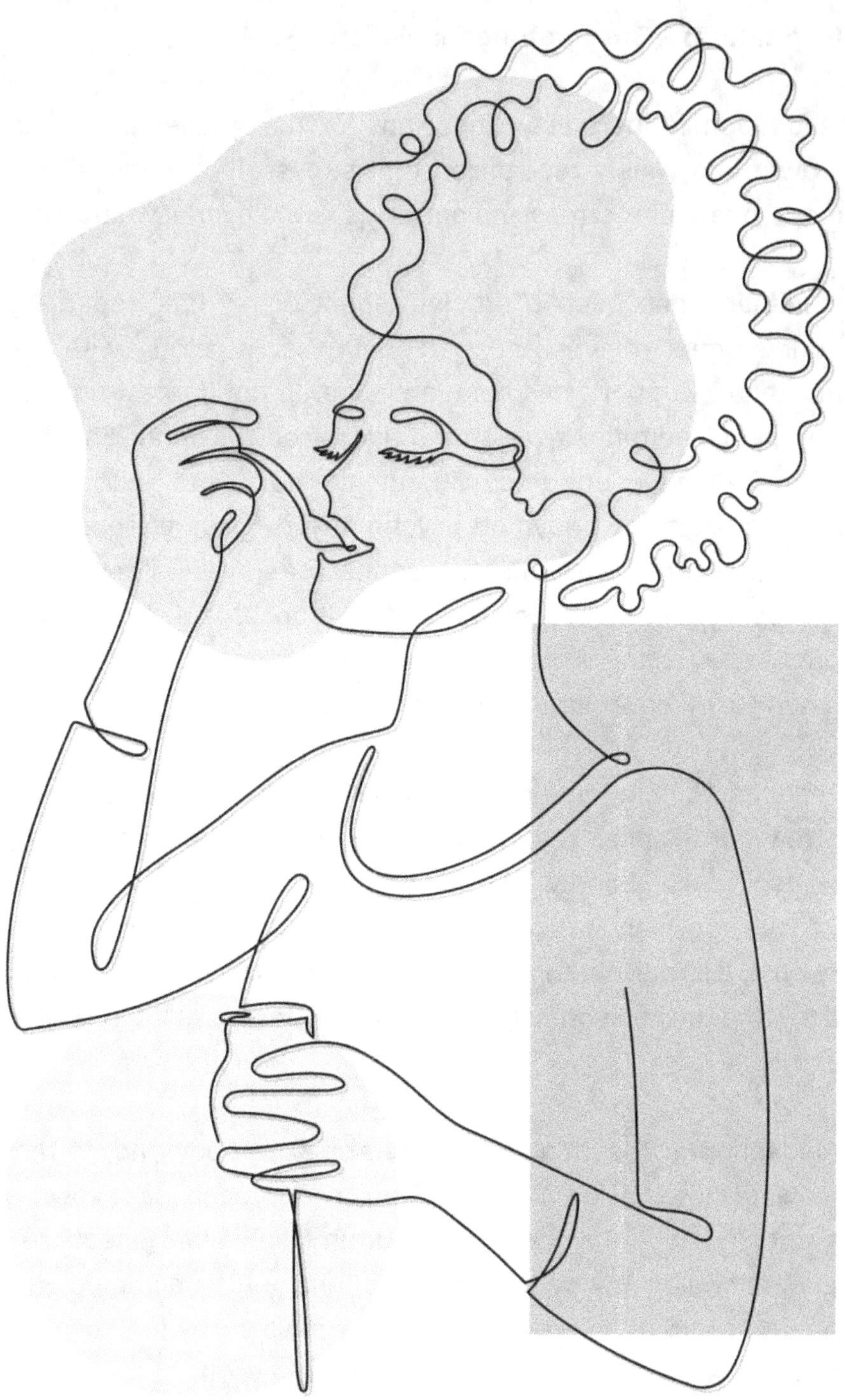

Meditation: A Cornerstone for Holistic Health

Meditation is incredibly important for hair preservation and growth. It's widely recognized that stress often leads to hair loss, so reducing stress and anxiety is key to overall well-being.

Meditation has been a crucial aspect of my life, especially during times of war and personal loss. It, along with my husband's support, has been a lifeline. In the darkest times, I turned to meditation to relax and give my body a break, knowing I couldn't have endured without it. The intensity of some situations left my body and psyche frayed, making meditation and the ability to self-reflect essential for survival. I'm grateful for having learned to meditate before it became a necessity; it provides stability in tumultuous and serene times alike, a means to discover inner peace amidst chaos.

The breadth of meditation is so vast it can hardly be confined to a few paragraphs. Yet, I choose to share because, for many years, I walked blindly, consuming the nonsense propagated in various books and articles. Fortuitous encounters with the right people, a strong personal desire, and extensive experience now allow me to shed some light on this topic for those interested in exploring it.

Meditation is essentially about relaxing the body and, in that relaxed state, using concentration to approach or resolve a particular issue. My meditations often involve introspection—understanding my reactions, emotions, and obstacles. It's about assuming full responsibility for my life; my feelings and fortunes are not dictated by others but by myself.

The relaxation process consists of two stages:

The first stage is finding "your breath," a comfortable rhythm unique to you during meditation. It took days for me to discover mine without any explicit instructions, but once found, it was unmistakable and ever-present.

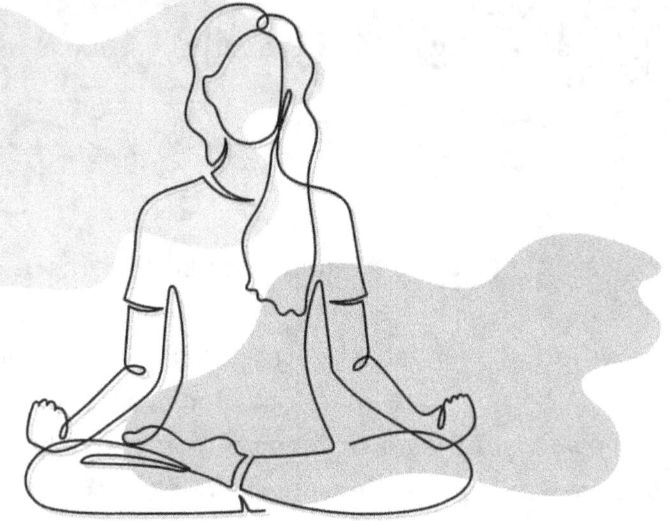

The second stage involves relaxing the body systematically from feet to head. Starting with the feet, gradually move your focus upward, allowing the stress mazes in your head to untangle themselves. This technique simplifies the entry into meditation.

Posture during meditation is important mainly to prevent dozing off, but comfort is key—no need to mimic others. My meditation journey began unorthodoxly, learning while walking, and now time, place, and activity don't impede my ability to meditate. It has become an inner state accessible anytime, anywhere. Nevertheless, I favor seated meditation with headphones and music for deep immersion.

In conclusion, there are four pivotal elements: physical activity, water, nutrition, and meditation. The first three pertain to the body, the last to the psyche. From this, we can derive a simple equation for life balance and well-being:

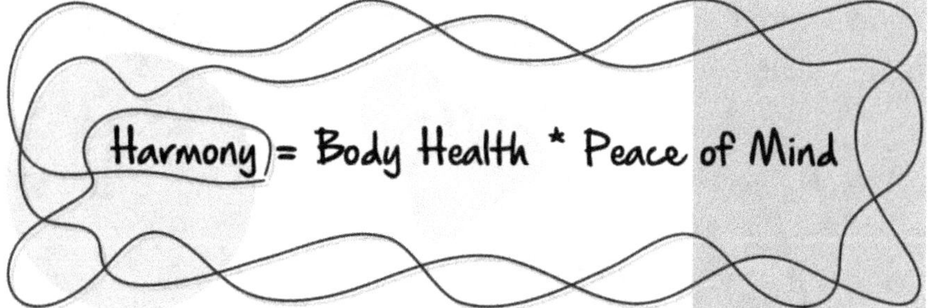

I have outlined methods that resonate with me, aligning with my preferences, and proving to be enjoyable and effortless. However, the approaches to maintaining bodily health and mental serenity are manifold. For example, someone might achieve a state akin to meditative clarity while running on a treadmill. Despite the physical exertion, they step away mentally rejuvenated.

The crux lies in pinpointing your own objectives. My meditation practice is centered around bodily relaxation, alleviating emotional stress, and uncovering answers to personal inquiries. Similarly, one could turn to various relaxation techniques, consult a therapist, or even keep a journal to fulfill these same needs.

Armed with the understanding of this formula, each individual has the capacity to discover their own unique strategies and paths to their goals. Often, the solutions lie within oneself — it's just a matter of engaging in self-dialogue.

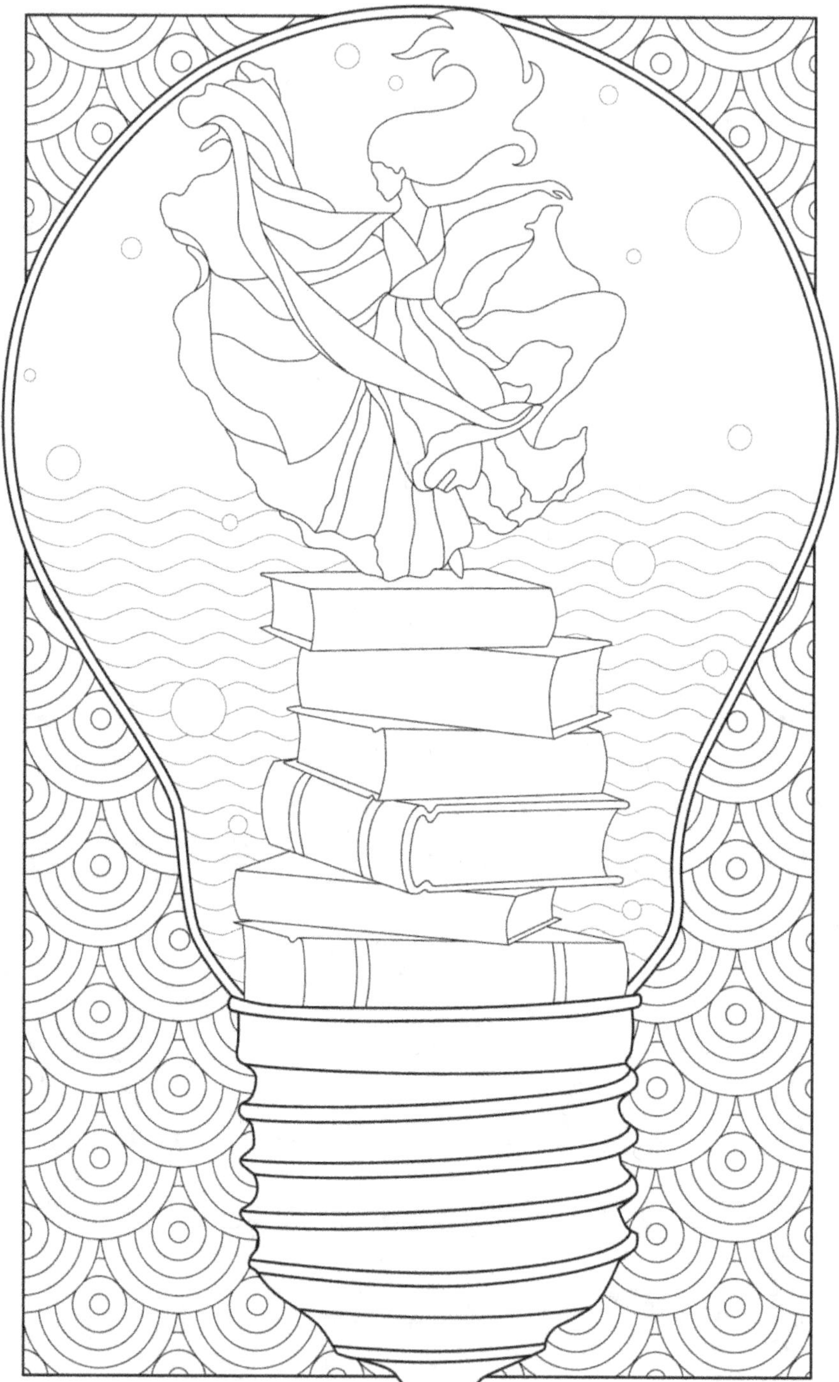

A Bit of Theory

Throughout my life, I've read numerous books on personal development and self-improvement. I vividly recall the often protracted introductions and explanations that spanned half the book. With that in mind, I approached this subject differently.

Practice comes first. These simple methods are for anyone to customize to their needs. The theoretical part, while explanatory, might not captivate everyone—only those intrigued by understanding the third formula and its interpretation.

Many years ago, a manager of a mid-sized company shared their experience with me. They had provided sales training with the expectation of improved performance. Initially, sales soared as the team sold with unprecedented enthusiasm. However, the spike in sales was short-lived, declining to prior levels and even lower. Upon reviewing the training materials at the manager's request, I analyzed them and extracted a formula that proved universally applicable to every action and situation I've since encountered:

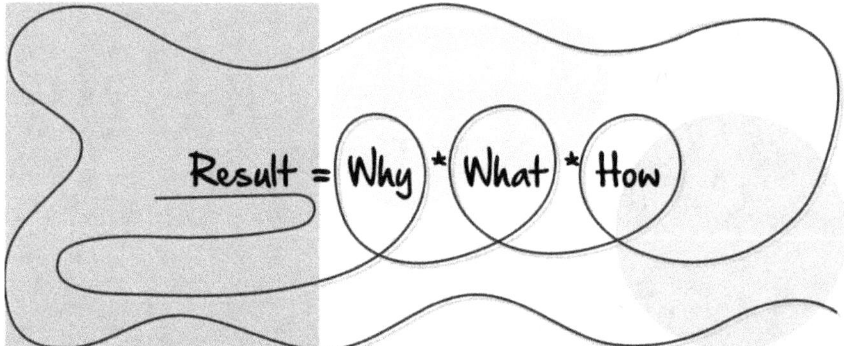

Mathematically, if any component of this equation is zero, the result is nil. That's precisely what transpired with the sales team—they lacked the "why." The training imparted knowledge on "what" to do and "how" to do it but failed to instill a reason to excel. Consequently, performance reverted to its original state.

Internal motivation is paramount, hence "why" leads the formula. If you picked up this guide, you're likely motivated to improve your hair's condition. Identifying your specific motivation—asking "Why do I want this?"—can offer profound self-insight. Dare to provide yourself with an honest answer, and you might discover much about your inner self.

I've detailed WHAT to do: massage. And I've explained HOW to do it: in my instance, with a hairbrush. You can use any tool you prefer, whether fingers, brushes, special scalp massagers, etc. Knowing your "why" equips you to commence your journey; with this, you have all the necessary information for results.

Let's now turn our attention to WHY and HOW the entire system operates, starting with the impact of massage, whether it be on the head, hand, or heel.

Massage: A Fundamental of Vitality

Consider our body akin to a sponge, a highly water-composed entity, flexible and porous. Massage operates on a simple mechanical principle akin to the sponge analogy. When pressure is applied to a sponge, water is expelled, and upon release, the sponge reabsorbs water. Massage mirrors this process in the human body.

The Ebb and Flow of Fluids: Applying pressure through massage sets bodily fluids in motion, transforming stagnant tissue pools into dynamic streams. This action creates a pressure gradient, inviting fresh fluids to occupy the vacated spaces. Blood, the life-giving fluid, rushes in, swelling the capillaries and delivering a bounty of oxygen and nutrients to each cell. Concurrently, the lymphatic system escalates its pace, carrying away waste. This is the dance of renewal—a rejuvenation of the body's landscapes.

The Hair's Life Cycle: To fully grasp massage's impact on hair, one must zoom in on the hair's existence. Picture the scalp, a bustling metropolis with roughly 100,000 hair citizens. Can you imagine maintaining peak productivity 24/7 for years, only pausing for a brief 3–4-month respite before resuming the cycle? This Herculean routine is the hair's standard modus operandi, broken down into three distinct phases.

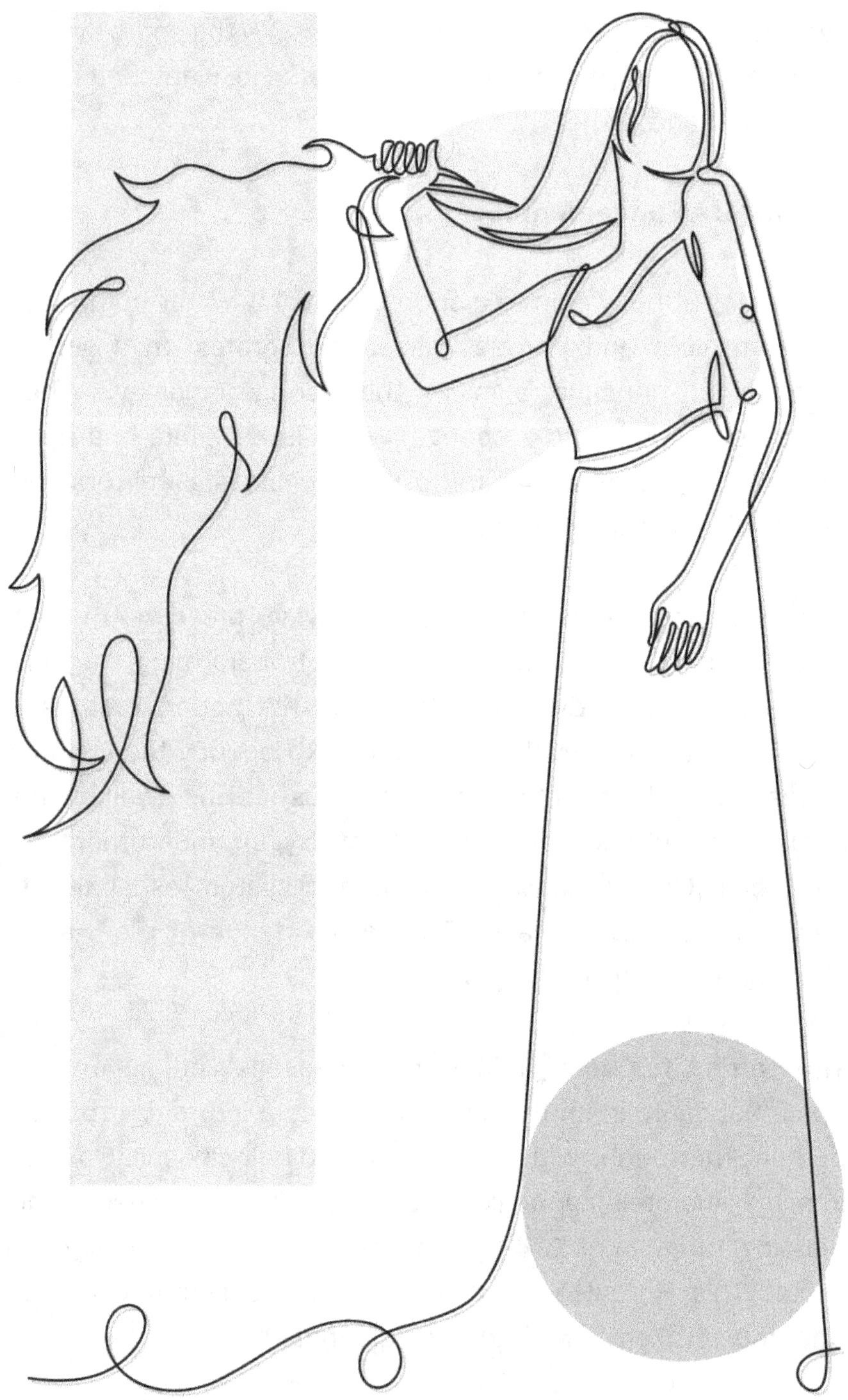

Phase 1

In our body's miraculous design, each of the roughly 100,000 hairs on the human head functions like a miniaturized, self-sufficient factory, with its own dedicated workforce:

The Growth Phase (Anagen): This phase can span 2 to 6 years and is largely determined by genetics. At the factory's core is the hair root, where new cells are produced, crafting the hair that surfaces about 1-1.5 cm each month.

The Raw Material Supplier: This is the blood supply, delivering essential nutrients to nurture the growth.

The Guard: A tiny muscle accompanies each hair, playing a key role in thermoregulation by adjusting the hair's position relative to the skin.

The Promotion Department: These are the melanin-producing cells, responsible for hair's pigment.

The Packaging Department: The sebaceous gland coats the hair in oils, contributing to its sheen and protection.

But the element that piqued my interest most is the hair's muscle, known as the arrector pili. In response to cold, it contracts, raising the hair to trap air for warmth. In heat, it relaxes, allowing the hair to lie flat and not insulate. When frightened or stressed, this muscle also contracts, a vestige of our fight or flight instincts, which in the animal kingdom, serves to make creatures appear larger to deter threats.

However, under intense or chronic stress, this muscle can constrict excessively, leading to premature hair shedding. The body, interpreting stress as a survival threat, conservatively halts non-essential functions like hair growth to conserve resources.

Thus, learning to relax and manage stress is not just a mental health issue; it's integral to physical health, including maintaining a full head of hair.

The more I studied the intricacies of a single hair, from its structure to its functions, the more I marveled at the body's complexity. It all circles back to safeguarding our most vital organ, the brain. If the brain is content to analyze and engage, the whole system, hair included, flourishes.

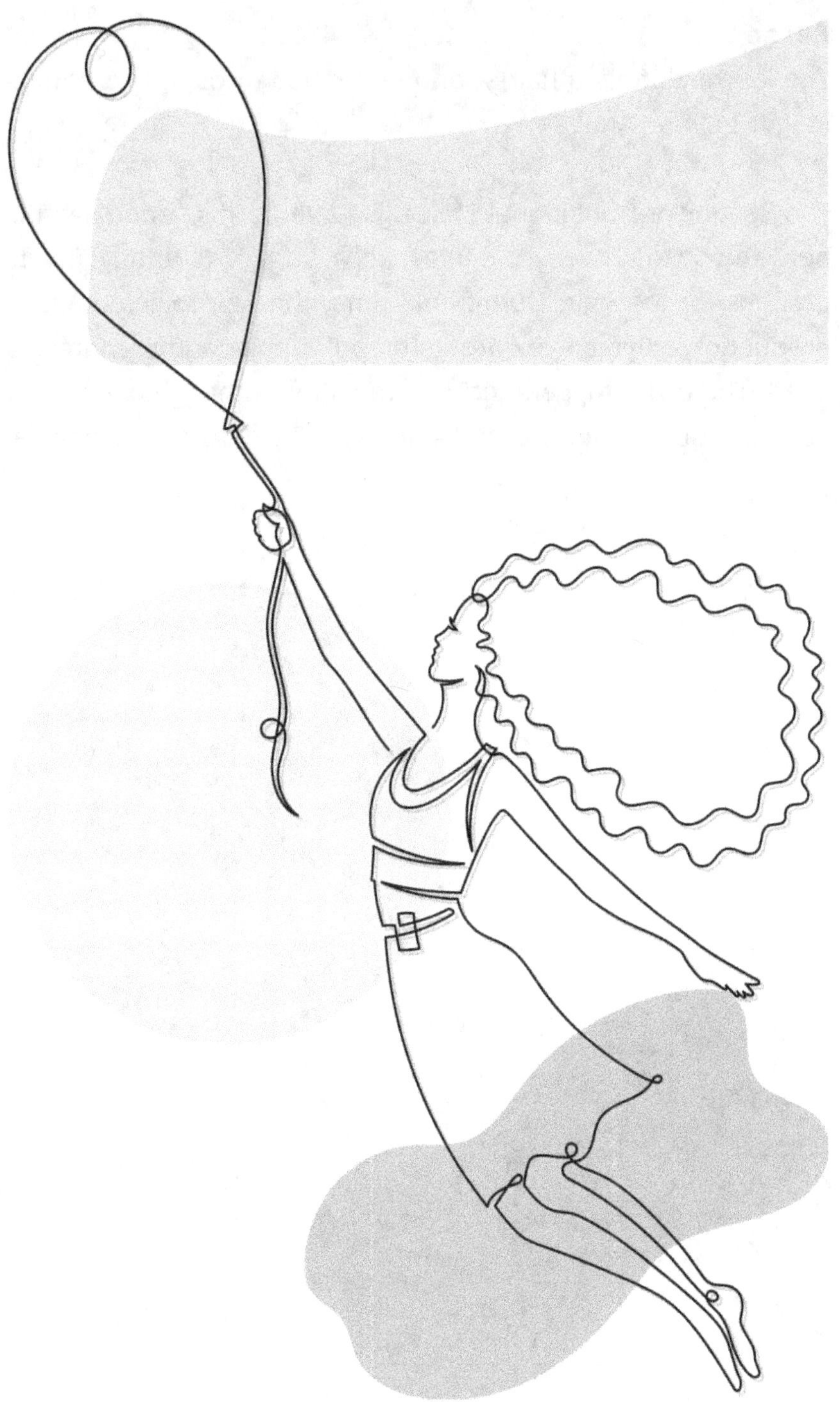

Phase 2

The journey of each hair strand continues through two critical stages beyond Anagen:

The Resting or Transitional Phase (Catagen): This period, lasting between 2 to 4 weeks, serves as a sort of 'shutting down' process for the hair. During this time, the hair follicle ceases production, severs ties with its blood supply, and prepares to shed. The exact triggers for this transition remain a mystery to science, but it's a natural progression in the hair's lifecycle.

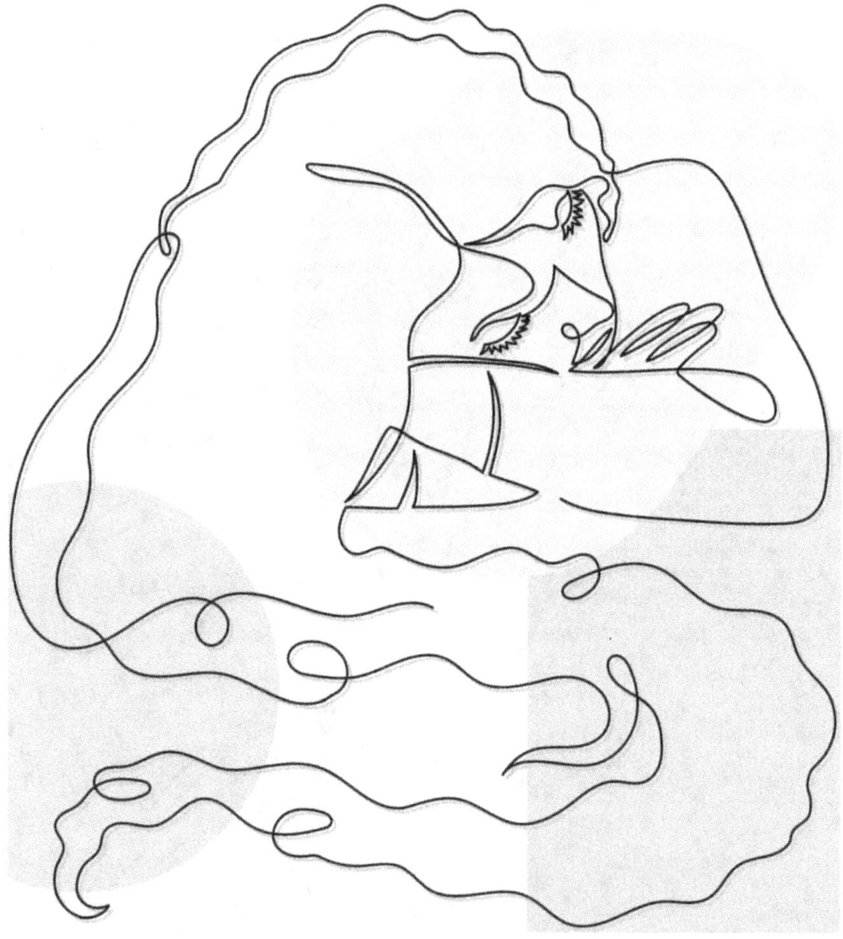

Phase 3

The Shedding Phase (Telogen): In this final phase, the hair strand exists in a state of rest for 2 to 4 months, awaiting its eventual departure from the scalp. This delay is why stress or illness-related hair loss isn't immediate; the impact unfolds gradually over time, often catching us by surprise weeks or months later.

The onset of increased hair loss post-massage puzzles many, but it's actually quite logical. Healthy, actively growing hairs aren't prone to shedding; they continue their lifecycle uninterrupted. It's the hairs in the Telogen phase—those already destined for shedding—that are expedited along by the massage. The process doesn't so much cause hair loss as it accelerates the departure of hairs that are already at the end of their cycle. From my personal experience, after the initial wave of shedding subsides, what follows is a period of stability and renewed growth, with minimal hair loss despite more vigorous and extended massage sessions.

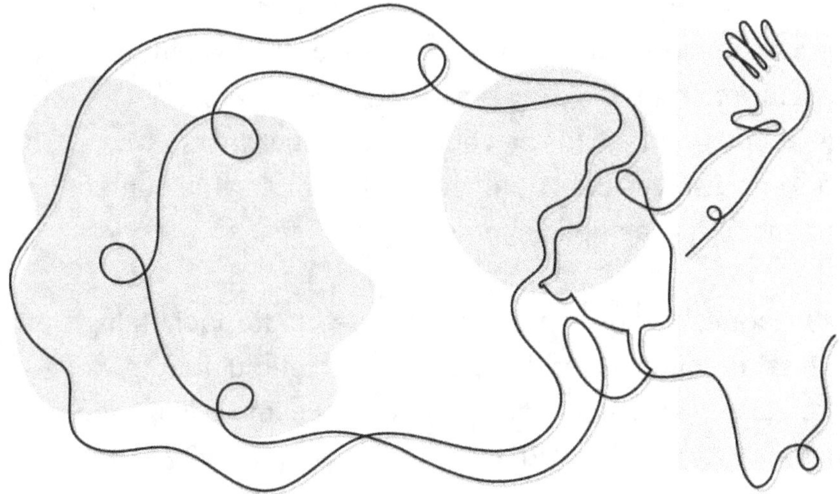

Sebaceous Gland: The Hair's Natural Armor

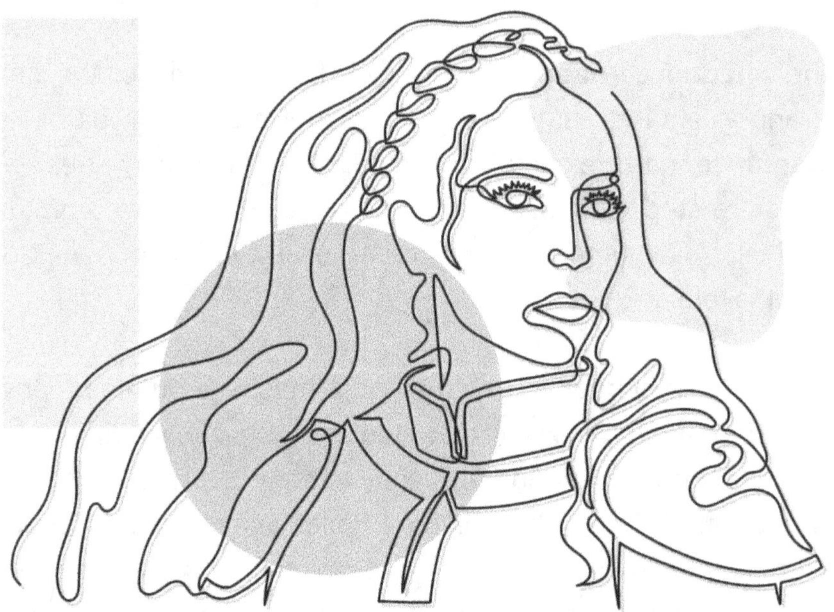

Every hair on our head, while primarily serving as a protective element, comes equipped with its own built-in defense mechanism, akin to a warrior's suit of armor. This defense is orchestrated by an individual sebaceous gland assigned to each hair, secreting sebum to coat the strand. This lipid layer not only acts as a shield but also imparts the glossy sheen that is often sought after in the hair care industry. Hence, I liken the sebaceous gland to a packaging department where the packaging serves dual purposes: safeguarding the content and enhancing its aesthetic appeal.

Consistent massage nurtures these glands, facilitating their natural function. Over time, as they are stimulated to work as intended by nature, the hair's appearance improves, becoming increasingly lustrous with each passing month.

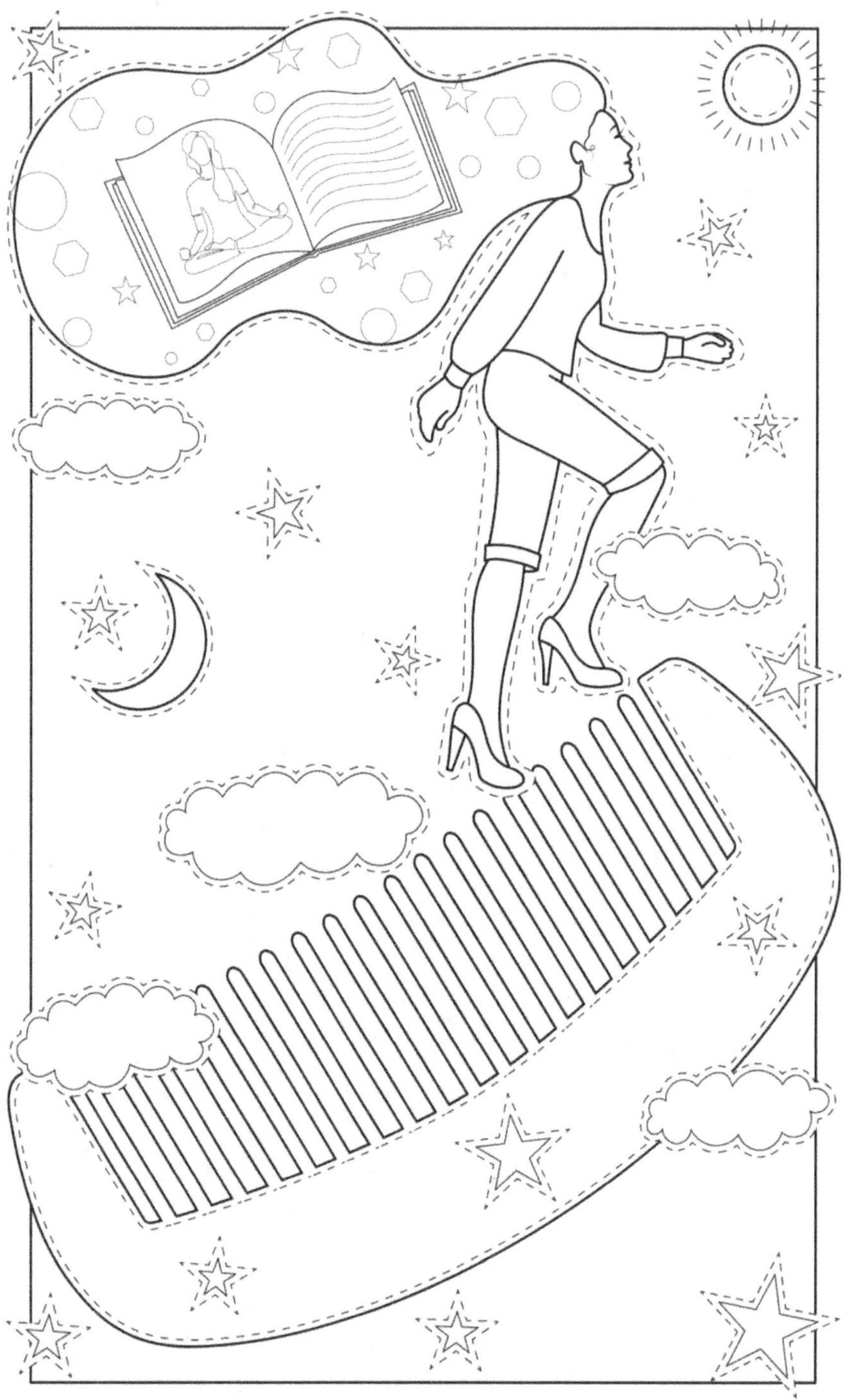

Afterword

With the practicalities, mechanisms, and philosophies explored, we arrive at a juncture of reflection.

Hair's Hierarchy of Needs: In the grand scheme of biological priorities, hair ranks below critical organs like the brain and heart. Our survival doesn't depend on luxurious locks. Thus, when resources are scarce, hair's nourishment takes a backseat.

Through scalp massage, we artfully redirect attention and nutrients to our hair, fostering its health and luster outside of the body's primary concerns.

Foundations First: Addressing cosmetic issues while neglecting fundamental health is akin to painting over a damaged façade. It's crucial to ensure the scalp is healthy before attempting to enhance hair through massage or other means. This perspective is drawn from my own experiences of sometimes leaping without looking, a reminder of the importance of foundational health.

The Essence of Self-Love: Contemplating self-love, I've discovered its essence isn't found in external wisdom but through inward journeying. Self-love, I've realized, means embracing my entirety, shedding undue guilt, and nurturing myself with attentive care. This revelation is deeply personal, and for each person, the understanding of self-love will be uniquely their own.

In closing, this book's message extends beyond hair care—it's a testament to the interplay of self-care, understanding, and the tender act of prioritizing oneself.

In using hair care as a microcosm of self-love, I've come to appreciate:

Forgiveness: I don't castigate myself for hair loss. Each moment in my life, I've acted with my best knowledge and abilities. With experience comes new methods and perspectives.

Acceptance: Embracing my current state, acknowledging that my hair isn't what it once was, propels me to change what I can without dwelling on regrets.

Patience: Recognizing that the body's changes are gradual yet responsive, I remind myself that progress is assured with persistent guidance and time.

Pleasure: The journey needs to be as pleasurable as it is effective. By infusing enjoyment into the process, I ensure it's a part of my life that I look forward to each day.

Consistency: Regularity is the cornerstone of success. The daily practice of massage, far from being burdensome, has become an effortless ritual.

Phrases like "Those who seek will find," "Where there's a will, there's a way," and "Onward and upward" resonate, yet the purpose of this book isn't to prescribe a single path but to offer a guide for those forging their own. It's here, within these pages, and within you—in the head and heart.

My wish is simple: Live fully, create joyfully, and remember that our world is crafted for love and happiness.

Thank you for joining me on this journey through the pages of my book. In it, I've woven threads of my experience and insights, all in the hopes of guiding you to a closer acquaintance with your inner self and to spark a renaissance for your hair.

Each reader's takeaway from a book is as distinct and extraordinary as they are. Your reflections are invaluable, not just to me but to the shared path we walk with others on similar quests.

If you feel moved to do so, I welcome you to share your thoughts and the resonance of this book with me and others by leaving a review. Your feedback is a gift I cherish and await with gratitude.

Thank you, once more, for your time and spirit.

PS

Maybe you have noticed line-art pictures in the beginning of each chapter. This is my gift for you. I've created them for those who wants to try one of the best relaxing and coming practices – coloring. Your movement to self-love may start here with easy and pleasant way:)

In case you would like to write me about your impression and results personally, address: lifeisforloveandjoy@gmail.com

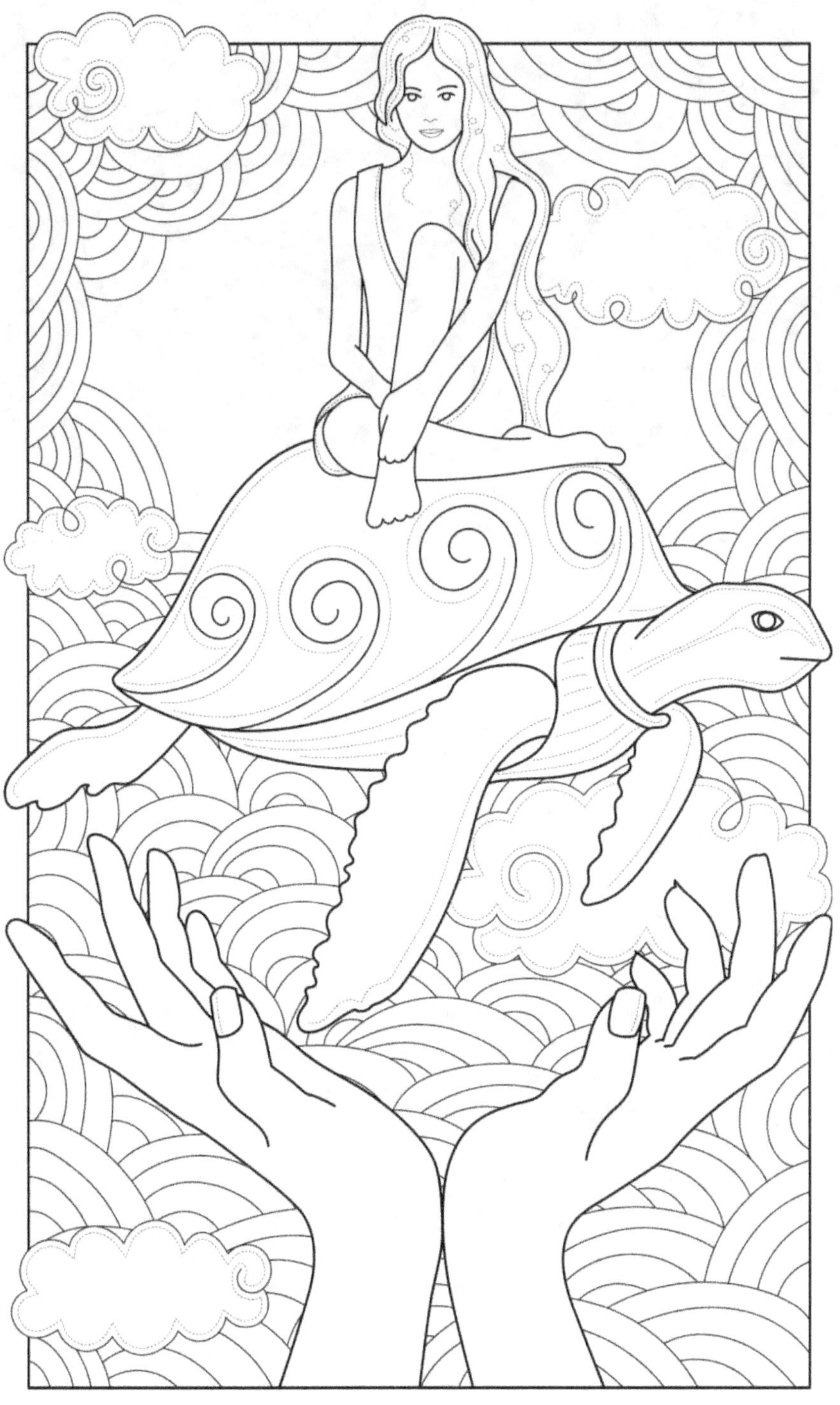

www.ingramcontent.com/pod-product-compliance
Lightning Source LLC
Chambersburg PA
CBHW070759250726
48662CB00004B/1888